Nephrology

Editor

PARVATHI PERUMAREDDI

PRIMARY CARE:
CLINICS IN OFFICE PRACTICE

www.primarycare.theclinics.com

Consulting Editor
JOEL J. HEIDELBAUGH

December 2020 • Volume 47 • Number 4

ELSEVIER

1600 John F. Kennedy Boulevard ⚫ Suite 1800 ⚫ Philadelphia, Pennsylvania, 19103-2899

http://www.theclinics.com

PRIMARY CARE: CLINICS IN OFFICE PRACTICE Volume 47, Number 4
December 2020 ISSN 0095-4543, ISBN-13: 978-0-323-76095-9

Editor: Katerina Heidhausen
Developmental Editor: Laura Fisher

Primary Care: Clinics in Office Practice (ISSN: 0095-4543) is published quarterly by Elsevier Inc., 360 Park Avenue South, New York, NY 10010-1710. Months of issue are March, June, September, and December. Periodicals postage paid at New York, NY and additional mailing offices. Subscription prices are $253.00 per year (US individuals), $538.00 (US institutions), $100.00 (US students), $303.00 (Canadian individuals), $609.00 (Canadian institutions), $100.00 (Canadian students), $357.00 (international individuals), $609.00 (international institutions), and $175.00 (international students). Foreign air speed delivery is included in all *Clinics* subscription prices. All prices are subject to change without notice. POSTMASTER: Send address changes to *Primary Care: Clinics in Office Practice*, Elsevier Periodicals Customer Service, 11830 Westline Industrial Drive, St. Louis, MO 63146. Customer Service Health Sciences Division, Subscription Customer Service, 3251 Riverport Lane, Maryland Heights, MO 63043. **Customer Service: 1-800-654-2452 (U.S. and Canada); 314-447-8871 (outside U.S. and Canada). Fax: 314-447-8029. E-mail: journalscustomerservice-usa@elsevier.com (for print support); journalsonlinesupport-usa@elsevier.com (for online support).**

Reprints. For copies of 100 or more, of articles in this publication, please contact the Commercial Reprints Department, Elsevier Inc., 360 Park Avenue South, New York, NY 10010-1710. Tel. 212-633-3874; Fax: 212-633-3820; E-mail: reprints@elsevier.com.

Primary Care: Clinics in Office Practice is covered in *MEDLINE/PubMed (Index Medicus)* and *EMBASE/ Excerpta Medica, Current Contents/Clinical Medicine, and ISI/BIOMED.*

Contributors

CONSULTING EDITOR

JOEL J. HEIDELBAUGH, MD, FAAFP, FACG
Clinical Professor, Departments of Family Medicine and Urology, Director of Medical Student Education and Clerkship Director, Department of Family Medicine, University of Michigan Medical School, Ann Arbor, Michigan, USA; Ypsilanti Health Center, Ypsilanti, Michigan, USA

EDITOR

PARVATHI PERUMAREDDI, DO
Assistant Professor of Family Medicine, Charles E. Schmidt College of Medicine, Florida Atlantic University, Boca Raton, Florida, USA

AUTHORS

OLTJON ALBAJRAMI, MD
Section of Nephrology, Department of Medicine, Boston Medical Center and Boston University School of Medicine, Boston, Massachusetts, USA

KATHERINE VOGEL ANDERSON, PharmD, BCACP
Associate Professor and PGY1 Residency Director, University of Florida College of Pharmacy, Gainesville, Florida, USA

REBECCA BEYTH, MD
Professor, Division of Internal Medicine, Associate Residency Program Director, University of Florida College of Medicine, NF/SG Veterans Health System GRECC, Gainesville, Florida, USA

KELLEY BISHOP, MD
Assistant Professor, Department of Family Medicine, University of Mississippi Medical Center, Jackson, Mississippi, USA

RYAN BONNER, MD
Department of Medicine, Boston Medical Center and Boston University School of Medicine, Boston, Massachusetts, USA

BRENDAN T. BOWMAN, MD
University of Virginia School of Medicine, Charlottesville, Virginia, USA

CORNELIA CHARLES, MD
Department of Veterans Affairs Medical Center, West Palm Beach, Florida, USA

GATES B. COLBERT, MD, FASN
Clinical Assistant Professor, Texas A&M College of Medicine, Dallas, Texas, USA

JIGAR CONTRACTOR, MD
Assistant Professor, Department of Medicine, Division of General Internal Medicine, Section of Hospital Medicine, Weill Cornell Medical College, New York, New York, USA

JOANNE DANNENHOFFER, MD, MS
Assistant Professor, Department of Family and Community Medicine, Albany Medical College, Albany, New York, USA

ALLISON H. FERRIS, MD
Associate Professor of Medicine, Charles E. Schmidt College of Medicine, Florida Atlantic University, Boca Raton, Florida, USA

JENNIFER G. FOSTER, MD, MBA, FACP
Assistant Professor of Medicine, Charles E. Schmidt College of Medicine, Florida Atlantic University, Boca Raton, Florida, USA

KEITH J. FOSTER, MD, MBA, CPE, FAAPMR
Clinical Affiliate Assistant Professor, Broward Health North, Deerfield Beach, Florida, USA

NIDA HAMIDUZZAMAN, MD, FACP
Clinical Associate Professor of Medicine, Division of Geriatric, Hospital, Palliative and General Internal Medicine, Keck School of Medicine of USC, Los Angeles, California, USA

JAMES HUDSPETH, MD
Department of Medicine, Boston Medical Center and Boston University School of Medicine, Boston, Massachusetts, USA

JACKCY JACOB, MD, FACP, FAAP
Assistant Professor, Department of Medicine, Albany Medical College, Albany, New York, USA

SANA F. KHAN, MBBS
University of Virginia School of Medicine, Charlottesville, Virginia, USA

ARAM KIM, MD
Assistant Professor, Department of Medicine, Division of General Internal Medicine, Section of Hospital Medicine, Weill Cornell Medical College, New York, New York, USA

PEROLA LAMBA, MD
Fellow, Department of Medicine, Division of Nephrology and Hypertension, Weill Cornell Medical College, New York, New York, USA

SAI SUDHA MANNEMUDDHU, MD, FAAP
Fellow, Department of Pediatrics, Division of Nephrology, University of Florida College of Medicine, Gainesville, Florida, USA

LISA C. MARTINEZ, MD
Charles E. Schmidt College of Medicine, Florida Atlantic University, Boca Raton, Florida, USA

TOBE MOMAH, MD
Assistant Professor, Department of Family Medicine, University of Mississippi Medical Center, Jackson, Mississippi, USA

KI HEON NAM, MD
Assistant Professor, Department of Internal Medicine, Division of Hospital Medicine, Yonsei University College of Medicine, Seoul, Republic of Korea

JASON C. OJEDA, MD, FACP
Primary Care Program Director, Assistant Professor of Medicine, Department of Internal Medicine, Thomas Jefferson University, Philadelphia, Pennsylvania, USA

PARVATHI PERUMAREDDI, DO
Assistant Professor of Family Medicine, Charles E. Schmidt College of Medicine, Florida Atlantic University, Boca Raton, Florida, USA

SETH ANTHONY POLITANO, DO, FACP
Clinical Associate Professor of Medicine, Division of Geriatric, Hospital, Palliative and General Internal Medicine, Keck School of Medicine of USC, Los Angeles, California, USA

JANET RICKS, DO
Professor, Program Director, Department of Family Medicine, University of Mississippi Medical Center, Jackson, Mississippi, USA

ANNIE RUTTER, MD, MS
Associate Professor, Department of Family and Community Medicine, Albany Medical College, Albany, New York, USA

RACHEL SHADDOCK, PharmD
PGY1 Pharmacy Resident, University of Florida College of Pharmacy, Gainesville, Florida, USA

DARIN P. TRELKA, MD, PhD
Assistant Professor of Pathology, Charles E. Schmidt College of Medicine, Florida Atlantic University, Boca Raton, Florida, USA

ASHISH UPADHYAY, MD
Section of Nephrology, Department of Medicine, Boston Medical Center and Boston University School of Medicine, Boston, Massachusetts, USA

ANJU YADAV, MD, FASN
Assistant Professor of Medicine, Division of Nephrology, Hypertension and Transplantation, Thomas Jefferson University, Philadelphia, Pennsylvania, USA

Contents

Foreword: "So Am I Leaking Pasta?"   xiii

Joel J. Heidelbaugh

Preface: xv

Parvathi Perumareddi

Approach to Electrolyte Abnormalities, Prerenal Azotemia, and Fluid Balance   555

Lisa C. Martinez, Sana F. Khan, and Brendan T. Bowman

> Volume and electrolyte evaluation and management is seen frequently in primary care practices. Some of the most common abnormalities encountered in outpatient practices are prerenal azotemia, dysnatremias, and altered potassium levels. Perturbations in volume or electrolyte concentrations can lead to serious organ dysfunction as well as hemodynamic collapse. This review focuses on the maintenance and regulation of intravascular volume and electrolytes, specifically sodium and potassium.

Acute Kidney Injury   571

Jackcy Jacob, Joanne Dannenhoffer, and Annie Rutter

> Acute kidney injury (AKI) is defined as an increase in serum creatinine or a decrease in urine output over hours to days. A thorough history and physical examination can help categorize the underlying cause as prerenal, intrinsic renal, or postrenal. Initial evaluation and management of AKI in the community setting includes laboratory work-up, medication adjustment, identification and reversal of underlying cause, and referral to appropriate specialty care. Even one episode of AKI increases the risk of cardiovascular disease, chronic kidney disease, and death. Therefore, early determination of etiology, management, and long-term follow-up of AKI are essential.

Chronic Kidney Disease   585

Cornelia Charles and Allison H. Ferris

> Chronic kidney disease is encountered by the primary care physician, in no small part owing to the high rates of hypertension and diabetes, the 2 most common etiologies of chronic kidney disease in the United States. As a primary care physician, it is important to understand the epidemiology, pathophysiology, and evaluation methods of chronic kidney disease even before a referral to nephrology. Additionally, the primary care physician plays a vital role in mitigating the risks of chronic kidney disease as well as the complications and comorbidities.

Nephrotic Syndrome   597

Seth Anthony Politano, Gates B. Colbert, and Nida Hamiduzzaman

> Nephrotic syndrome is one cause of end-stage kidney disease. Because edema is a common presenting feature and hypertension and dyslipidemia

are often present in nephrotic syndrome, it is important for the primary care physician to suspect this entity. Common causes in adults include diabetic nephropathy, focal segmental glomerulosclerosis, and membranous nephropathy. In adults, many primary causes are due to an underlying disease. A cause of the nephrotic syndrome should be established with serologic workup and renal consultation. Renal biopsy is necessary in those with an unknown cause to or classify disease. Treatment focuses on symptoms, complications, and the primary cause.

Nephritic Syndrome   615

Perola Lamba, Ki Heon Nam, Jigar Contractor, and Aram Kim

Nephritic syndrome is a constellation of hematuria, proteinuria, hypertension, and in some cases acute kidney injury and fluid retention characteristic of acute glomerulonephritis. Infection-related glomerulonephritis, IgA nephropathy, lupus nephritis, membranoproliferative glomerulonephritis, and antineutrophil cytoplasmic antibody–associated vasculitis are the most common diseases in nephritic syndrome that primary care physicians might encounter in practice such that a solid comprehension of these can lead to earlier detection. This article describes the pathophysiology, incidence, clinical presentation, treatment, and disease progression of these nephritic syndrome entities, and provides guidance for when to refer to a nephrologist.

Renovascular Hypertension   631

Sai Sudha Mannemuddhu, Jason C. Ojeda, and Anju Yadav

Renovascular hypertension (RVH) is relatively common but underrecognized cause of resistant hypertension in clinical practice. Most patients with RVH have suboptimal control of hypertension in spite of being on multiple anti hypertensive medications. Prompt diagnosis and management is crucial to prevent long term morbidity and mortality. Initial evaluation by primary care physicians can expedite this to improve patient outcomes by co-managing hypertension specialists. In addition to pharmacologic and nonpharmacologic measures, some patients may benefit from angioplasty. This article discusses various definitions of hypertension, approach to diagnosis of RVH, and management. Data from clinical trials are discussed with evidence-based medicine practice recommendations.

Diabetic Kidney Disease   645

Ryan Bonner, Oltjon Albajrami, James Hudspeth, and Ashish Upadhyay

Diabetic kidney disease (DKD) is the most common cause of chronic kidney disease in the United States. Approximately 30% to 40% of individuals with diabetes mellitus develop DKD, and the presence of DKD significantly elevates the risk for morbidity and mortality. Understanding of DKD has grown in recent years. This review describes the pathogenesis of DKD and expands on evidence-based strategies for DKD management, integrating traditional approaches for hyperglycemia, hypertension, and albuminuria management with emerging therapeutic options. Given the public health burden of DKD, it is essential to prioritize prevention, recognition, and management of DKD in the primary care setting.

Nephrolithiasis   661

Kelley Bishop, Tobe Momah, and Janet Ricks

> Nephrolithiasis, commonly known as kidney stones, may be localized to any part of the urothelial system, causing common systemic symptoms, some of which may become acute. Primary care physicians increasingly are the first line of management for this condition, making recognition and prompt treatment essential. This article highlights the pathogenesis of kidney stones, the risk factors for their formation, and common complications. The article concludes with management guidelines for nephrolithiasis and when primary care physicians should refer patients to nephrology or urology. In light of the current opioid epidemic, salient points for nonopioid treatment as initial treatment of nephrolithiasis likewise are discussed.

Autosomal Dominant Polycystic Kidney Disease   673

Parvathi Perumareddi and Darin P. Trelka

> Autosomal Dominant Polycystic Kidney Disease is an inherited multisystemic disorder of the renal tubules with subsequent formation of multiple cysts and enlargement of the kidney, affecting various organs. Diagnosis is initially suspected in those with family history and/or individuals who develop hypertension early on (secondary hypertension) or certain symptoms. Renal function is initially preserved for years secondary to compensatory mechanisms. Associated conditions include: liver cysts, berry aneurysms, kidney stones, etc. The disease course is variable, but patients often progress to end-stage renal failure by age 60. There is no known cure, however, risk factor modification at early stages is critical. Renal transplant is the optimal treatment in ESRD.

Renal Repercussions of Medications   691

Rachel Shaddock, Katherine Vogel Anderson, and Rebecca Beyth

> Medications are a common cause of acute kidney injury and chronic kidney disease. Older patients with multiple comorbidities and polypharmacy are at increased risk and require extra diligence. Antimicrobials, antihypertensives, and nonsteroidal anti-inflammatory drugs are common offenders of drug-induced kidney injury. Other drug classes that can cause kidney damage include immunosuppressive medications, statins, proton pump inhibitors, and herbal supplements. Awareness of such medications and their mechanisms of nephrotoxicity helps decrease morbidity and mortality. If nephrotoxic agents cannot be avoided, hydration, avoiding concomitant nephrotoxic medications, and using the lowest effective dose for the shortest duration are strategies that can decrease risk of kidney damage.

Care of the Renal Transplant Patient   703

Jennifer G. Foster and Keith J. Foster

> Renal transplant has become a mainstay of treatment of patients with chronic renal failure. With improving survival outcomes, primary care physicians should be informed of the nuances that come with the ongoing care

of this population and feel empowered to take part in the multidisciplinary care of these patients. This article provides an overview of the renal transplant process from initial evaluation through surgery and then focuses on long-term issues that renal transplant patients face in the primary care setting.

PRIMARY CARE:
CLINICS IN OFFICE PRACTICE

FORTHCOMING ISSUES

March 2021
Immigrant Health
Fern R. Hauck and Carina Brown,
Editors

June 2021
LGBTQ+ Health
Jessica Lapinski and Kristine Diaz, *Editors*

September 2021
Common Pediatric Issues in Primary Care
Luz M. Fernandez and Jonathan Becker,
Editors

RECENT ISSUES

September 2020
Immunizations
Margot Savoy, *Editor*

June 2020
Adolescent Medicine
Benjamin Silverberg, *Editor*

March 2020
Sports Medicine
Peter J. Carek, *Editor*

SERIES OF RELATED INTEREST

Medical Clinics (http://www.medical.theclinics.com)
Immunology & Allergy Clinics (https://www.immunology.theclinics.com)

THE CLINICS ARE AVAILABLE ONLINE!
Access your subscription at:
www.theclinics.com

Foreword
"So Am I Leaking Pasta?"

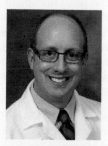

Joel J. Heidelbaugh, MD, FAAFP, FACG
Consulting Editor

Like many organs, the science of the kidney has always fascinated me and has provided a constant challenge in solving the enigmatic mystery of its many functions. As my wife is a pharmacist, I am constantly challenged to consider the renal excretion of drugs and how declining function impacts metabolism and excretion. Of course, this challenge is never mastered, which keeps me motivated to keep learning.

As an educator of students, residents, and especially patients, I've learned over the years to try to keep things as simple as possible. This translates to an insatiable quest to make analogies that people will understand and remember relative to pathophysiology. A common attempt at this practice often includes my analogy of how the kidney works as a filter. When I explain the concept of proteinuria, I explain how the kidney is a very smart filter that knows how much water and salt to keep versus how much to get rid of through the urine. Then, I explain how proteins are larger molecules that should not pass through the kidney and should be recirculated through the bloodstream, yet if they are excreted in significant quantity, then this may represent several forms of kidney damage and declining renal function. I use the analogy of making pasta in a large pot of boiling water, putting the strainer in the sink, then pouring the contents of the pot into the strainer with the goal of having the strainer retain the pasta and not leak through the strainer. The concept here is that the pasta is the protein (yes, I know it's a carbohydrate...) in my analogy. Then, of course, you eat the pasta and it circulates throughout the body. Sometimes my analogies are "lost in translation," and patients (and learners) think that what I'm trying to convey relative to kidney disease is that the patient is urinating pasta...

This issue of *Primary Care: Clinics in Office Practice* dedicated to nephrology serves as a contemporary primer for clinicians and learners at all stages in medical education for reviewing salient components of basic science, differential diagnosis, and clinical application of therapeutics for renal diseases. Articles dedicated to electrolytes, acute kidney injury, and chronic kidney disease provide information that can be used in daily

Prim Care Clin Office Pract 47 (2020) xiii–xiv
https://doi.org/10.1016/j.pop.2020.09.002
0095-4543/20/© 2020 Published by Elsevier Inc.

primarycare.theclinics.com

ambulatory and hospital-based practices. As rates of resistant hypertension increase, primary care clinicians can learn from the strategies in these articles to achieve appropriate blood pressure goals and minimize risk of renal disease. Additional articles on nephrotic and nephritic syndromes, polycystic kidney disease, diabetic nephropathy, and nephrolithiasis provide guideline-based approaches to cost-effective care. The issue ends with an excellent article dedicated to care of the renal transplant patient that will aid the primary care clinician in comanagement of these complex patients.

I am indebted to Dr Perumareddi and her talented authors for crafting very meaningful articles that review basic science applications and provide practical guidance for managing common and complex renal diseases. I hope that our readers will find this issue to be both informative and timely. I also hope that you enhance your understanding of renal function and create better analogies than I have!

Joel J. Heidelbaugh, MD, FAAFP, FACG
Departments of Family Medicine and Urology
University of Michigan Medical School
Ann Arbor, MI, USA

Ypsilanti Health Center
200 Arnet, Suite 200
Ypsilanti, MI 48198, USA

E-mail address:
jheidel@umich.edu

Preface

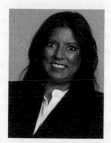

Parvathi Perumareddi, DO
Editor

An estimated 40 million individuals in the United States have kidney disease according to the National Institute of Diabetes and Digestive Kidney Diseases, with an estimated 1 in 3 individuals at risk. Recent statistics reveal that there are close to 100,000 people on a list for kidney transplant per United Network of Organ Sharing with an average wait time of 3.6 years.

Interestingly, although the kidneys filter approximately 200 quarts of blood daily, and also function to control blood pressure, manufacture red blood cells, and maintain bone health, upon insult, symptoms may not appear for years or sometimes even decades, which is why it is known as a "silent disease"; when present, the symptoms are often nonspecific, occasionally making diagnosis inconspicuous initially. In addition, the sources of renal injury are many and multifactorial, encompassing a wide range from genetic causes to medications to environmental/lifestyle factors to comorbid conditions, the latter including hypertension and diabetes. Chronic kidney disease, in particular is known to occur concomitantly with, and in association with cardiovascular disease. Furthermore, kidney disease can present early in life, affecting the spectrum of ages from the pediatric population through geriatrics. Renal diseases vary in acuity and chronicity as well as in progression of damage and breadth of symptoms.

Living with chronic renal disease can be very cumbersome for patients, affecting their quality of life. If untreated, kidney disease has the potential to lead to serious consequences, including end-stage renal disease or kidney failure, ultimately requiring dialysis or renal transplantation.

Kidney disease is ubiquitous, such that physicians of various specialties and fields often encounter patients with some variation or form of renal impairment. Prior to the patient reaching the nephrologist, it is likely the primary care physician who may have the first opportunity to detect and begin the workup and initial treatment for kidney disease. As such, understanding the various facets of kidney disease is vital as is keeping abreast of the latest advances in diagnosis and management.

My experience in renal disease began via my practice experience treating large numbers of patients with hypertension and diabetes through metabolic syndrome,

Prim Care Clin Office Pract 47 (2020) xv–xvi
https://doi.org/10.1016/j.pop.2020.09.001
0095-4543/20/© 2020 Published by Elsevier Inc.

primarycare.theclinics.com

many often having abnormal kidney function laboratory results. The prevention of complications from these disease states became one of my passions in medicine and a focus for my education for patients and now students.

Once I became involved in national recruitment studies at the VA surrounding blood pressure and proteinuria, the true prevalence and burden of kidney disease struck me. After leaving the VA practice and subsequently transitioning to a career in academic medicine, I became the course director for the Renal block in basic sciences for second-year medical students. This deeper immersion in nephrology over the past several years further piqued my interest in nephrology, but it was also the recent discovery that one of my best friends has end-stage renal disease and is awaiting a kidney transplant that heightened my curiosity in this field and ignited my drive to learn more.

It is an honor to present this special issue of Nephrology, illuminating not only the pathogenesis of a spectrum of common renal diseases but also the latest advances in therapy. This collection of articles was written by talented and experienced academic physicians across the country, ranging from family medicine and internal medicine/hospital medicine to pathology, nephrology, and transplant nephrology. My sincere and humble thanks go to each and every one of the authors for their time, conscientiousness, and diligence in writing articles providing integral information in an organized manner for the reader to absorb each facet of the disease from background, pathogenesis, presentation, workup, and management through referral to Nephrology. As we all face the uncertainty of the COVID pandemic, an unprecedented public health crisis, of which we do not yet fully understand the long-term effects, on a personal note, I would be remiss if I did not reflect upon and express my deepest gratitude to my mentors, without whom I would not be who I am today, not only as a physician but also as an educator, mentor, author, colleague, and person.

These two special mentors are my residency director, Dr. Diane K. Beebe, and my dad, Dr. Jayarama R. Perumareddi. During their careers, they dedicated their lives and time limitlessly as educators to countless numbers of students and as professors in their respective fields of family medicine and chemistry, both also having a deep and profound impact on me, contributing to my growth, professionally and personally. Dr. Beebe taught me how knowledge, a strong work ethic, communication, understanding, and compassion can make a long-lasting positive difference in our patients' lives and that of our students. She continues to motivate, encourage and support me today 20 plus years later, now as my dear friend.

My dad has inspired me throughout my life not only with his curiosity for knowledge and altruistic commitment to education, teaching, and scholarly work, but also through his steadfastness of character, integrity, empathy, and humility, which he has always exemplified, and which is valuable, now more than ever.

Along with Dr. Joel Heidelbaugh, whom I thank for this meaningful opportunity to serve as guest editor, it is my genuine and humble hope that you find this special issue most helpful in further stimulating your interest in and expanding your knowledge of nephrology in the care and treatment of your patients. Thank you.

Parvathi Perumareddi, DO
Florida Atlantic University
Schmidt College of Medicine
777 Glades Road
Boca Raton, FL 33431, USA

E-mail address:
pperumar@health.fau.edu

Approach to Electrolyte Abnormalities, Prerenal Azotemia, and Fluid Balance

Lisa C. Martinez, MD[a],*, Sana F. Khan, MBBS[b],
Brendan T. Bowman, MD[b]

KEYWORDS

- Prerenal azotemia • Hyponatremia • Hypernatremia • Hyperkalemia • Hypokalemia

KEY POINTS

- The approach to hypovolemic states and prerenal azotemia involves assessing cause and severity.
- Managing hypernatremia and hyponatremia depends on determining underlying cause.
- Hyperkalemia is relatively uncommon; however, hypokalemia is managed by cues from clinical presentation.

INTRODUCTION

The kidney serves several important functions in the human body including maintenance and regulation of fluid and electrolytes; excretion of metabolic and foreign substances, and hormone production including renin, erythropoietin, and 1,25 dihydroxyvitamin D.[1] Ideal function of many organs and cells is achieved by ensuring adequate volume status, acid-base balance, as well as maintaining sodium, potassium, and calcium levels in a very narrow range. Perturbations in any of these states can lead to serious organ dysfunction as well as hemodynamic collapse. This article focuses on the maintenance and regulation of intravascular volume and electrolytes, specifically sodium and potassium.

VOLUME REGULATION AND ASSESSMENT

Total body water is composed of extracellular volume (ECV) and intracellular volume (ICV), with approximately one-third composing the former and two-thirds the latter.[2]

[a] Florida Atlantic University, Charles E. Schmidt College of Medicine, 777 Glades Road, Boca Raton, FL 33431, USA; [b] University of Virginia School of Medicine, 1300 Jefferson Park Avenue, Charlottesville, VA 22903, USA
* Corresponding author.
E-mail address: lmartinez@health.fau.edu

Prim Care Clin Office Pract 47 (2020) 555–569
https://doi.org/10.1016/j.pop.2020.07.001
primarycare.theclinics.com

The ECV can be further broken down into the interstitial and plasma volume compartments, which make up approximately 60% and 17% of the ECV, respectively. Effective arterial circulating volume is primarily regulated by sensors in the afferent arterioles of the kidney, carotid sinus, and atria/ventricles of the heart.[3,4] Defense of volume status requires sodium retention—the main determinant of extracellular volume—and water reabsorption. In the kidney, the renin angiotensin aldosterone system (RAS) is activated to retain sodium. The ultimate generation of aldosterone, and its physiologic function, occur as follows:

- Renin, produced in the juxtaglomerular apparatus as a response to decreased renal perfusion, cleaves angiotensinogen to angiotensin I.
- Angiotensin I is converted to angiotensin II by circulating angiotensin-converting enzyme (ACE).
- Angiotensin II (and/or hyperkalemia) directly stimulates production of aldosterone in the zona glomerulosa of the adrenal glands.
- Angiotensin II and aldosterone promote sodium reabsorption and hence increased extracellular volume.[1,5]

Antidiuretic hormone (ADH), or arginine vasopressin, drives water reabsorption (and to some extent urea) in the collecting ducts of the nephron. ADH release is tightly regulated to maintain normal serum osmolality (280–290 mOsm/L), and its release is carefully governed by osmoreceptors in the hypothalamus.[6] In states of extremely low ECV, ADH release may be stimulated by baroreceptors/volume contraction.[7] This initiates a chain of events leading to water channel (aquaporin) insertion in the collecting duct and osmosis-driven reabsorption of water.[8]

Volume depletion has many causes, including acute blood loss, gastrointestinal (GI), renal or insensible losses, or decreased intake. The initial assessment of patients with hypovolemia includes a thorough history and examination. Patients may report typical histories of fluid loss such as diarrhea, vomiting, bleeding, fever, or decreased oral intake. Symptoms related to decreased tissue perfusion may also be present, such as postural dizziness, fatigue, chest pain, decreased urine output, or confusion. Postural hypotension, defined as a drop in systolic blood pressure of more than 20 mm Hg or 10 mm Hg drop in diastolic pressure, is a traditional tool for volume assessment but may be confounded by several factors such as examiner technique or the presence of autonomic dysfunction seen in long-standing diabetic neuropathy and parkinsonism. Postural dizziness and postural pulse increment of greater than or equal to 30/min have good sensitivity and specificity (97% and 98%, respectively) for blood loss greater than or equal to 630 mL but, however, do not perform as well for other causes of hypovolemia (sensitivity 43% and specificity 75%).[9,10] Other signs of hypovolemia include dry mucous membranes with tongue furrows, prolonged capillary refill, and dry axilla. However, many of these clinical findings have low sensitivity and specificity. Laboratory evaluation, most commonly blood urea nitrogen, creatinine, and serum and urine electrolytes, often accompanies the clinical examination to improve the diagnostic accuracy for a patient with suspected hypovolemia. Future office-based assessment tools for volume evaluation may include point-of-care ultrasound assessment or portable bioimpedance devices; however, none of these have been widely adopted in the ambulatory setting to date.[11] Patients with conditions of decreased effective circulating volume, such as acute decompensated heart failure or end-stage liver disease, are particularly difficult to diagnose. For example, the clinical sign of lower extremity edema correlates poorly with degree of heart failure and overall volume status.[12,13]

PRERENAL AZOTEMIA

Blood urea nitrogen (BUN) is a byproduct of protein break down and formed from metabolism of amino acids in the liver. Urea is normally reabsorbed constitutively in the ascending limb of the loop of Henle and the inner medullary collecting duct via specialized urea transporters. In states of hypovolemia and decreased effective circulating volume, ADH release increases renal reabsorption of urea and eventually elevated serum BUN.[14] Creatinine, a byproduct of muscle creatine, has a fairly stable turnover and is excreted but not reabsorbed in the kidney, making it a better marker of glomerular filtration rate (GFR) than BUN. The median BUN:creatinine ratio (measured in mg/dL) in a healthy individual is typically 15:1.[15] However, when renal blood flow is decreased, BUN is reabsorbed at a greater rate, with stable excretion of creatinine, resulting in elevation of the BUN:creatinine ratio, typically greater than 20:1.[15,16] This laboratory finding is termed "prerenal azotemia" and should be differentiated from the clinical syndrome of uremia. In prerenal azotemia, the drop in urinary urea excretion leads to a lower fractional excretion of urea and can be useful in differentiating prerenal states from intrinsic acute kidney injury. When calculating the fractional excretion of urea (FE_{UN}), a value less than 35% indicates a prerenal state. This FE_{UN} may be superior to the fractional excretion of sodium, especially in those taking diuretics.[17,18] It is important to note that a BUN:creatinine ratio greater than or equal to 20:1 may be seen in other conditions that result in increased urea production or decreased excretion (**Fig. 1**). These include GI bleeding, increased catabolic states, glucocorticoid administration, and excess protein ingestion.[14,19]

Treatment of hypovolemia or decreased effective circulating volume includes diagnosis and treatment of the underlying cause. If true intravascular volume depletion is diagnosed, then replacing volume with either oral hydration or intravenous fluids (IVFs) is indicated. Usually patients with modest symptoms of hypovolemia, yet adequate peripheral perfusion, may be treated as outpatients if they tolerate oral fluids and the source of volume loss can be controlled. Choice of oral hydration depends on the fluid loss and severity. In cases of diarrhea, if the patient is a healthy adult, recommendations to keep up with fluid losses through typical fluids (eg, watered down fruit juices/sports drinks, soups/broths) are usually sufficient. However, for patients with severe diarrhea, the very young or elderly, balanced oral rehydration solutions with sodium of 60 to 75 mEq/L and glucose of 75 to 90 mmol/L (equivalent in tonicity to "half normal saline") are ideal and available over the counter and at pharmacies.[20] **Table 1**

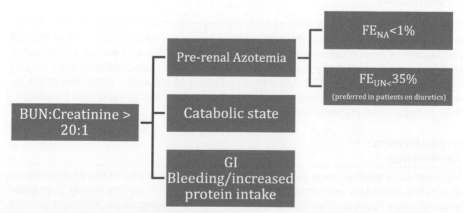

Fig. 1. Causes of increased BUN:creatinine ratio.

Table 1
Treatment of hypovolemia

Iso-osmolar Fluid Losses (Diarrhea, Vomiting, Diuretic Use, etc.)		
Mild-Moderate Without Signs of Hemodynamic Compromise and/or Comorbidities	Moderate but with Comorbidities, Very Young or Advanced Age	Severe with Hemodynamic Compromise

Young, healthy:
• Watered down fruit juice, sports drinks
• Soups/broths
	Oral replacement therapy
	• Hypo-osmolar fluids with equal parts of sodium and carbohydrates
	• Over-the-counter examples of premixed solutions include Pedialyte, Infalyte, or Resol
	• Packets are available but must be mixed with the correct amount of water to be effective
		Inpatient evaluation and treatment
		IVF
		• Metabolic alkalosis from vomiting or diuretic use
		  ○ 0.9% NaCl
		• Metabolic acidosis from GI losses
		  ○ Lactated Ringer solution

summarizes approach to treatment. To avoid hypovolemia and muscle cramping during exercise, athletes have historically been advised to proactively drink fluids; however, there is little basis for this recommendation and, in fact, there is risk of exercise-associated hyponatremia.[21] Most athletes can achieve adequate hydration by maintaining regular access to water and drinking to thirst. Addition of carbohydrates and/or electrolytes is not typically necessary for exercise less than 1 hour.[22]

Patients who cannot tolerate oral rehydration, or who have symptoms of decreased peripheral perfusion, should be observed in the hospital and administered IVFs. Most cases of volume depletion result in isoosmolar losses (eg, diarrhea), and choice of IVFs should be tailored to the presenting clinical scenario. For example, patients with non-gap acidosis due to GI losses should receive a balanced (eg, lactated ringers) or alkaline resuscitation fluid, whereas diuretic induced alkalosis with volume depletion responds well to normal saline (see **Table 1**).

DYSNATREMIAS

The kidney is the major regulator of both plasma sodium/osmolality and volume control. The former is controlled through variable water excretion and the latter through modulation of sodium excretion. By controlling water intake and excretion, the osmoregulatory system normally prevents the plasma sodium concentration from varying outside its normal range (136–145 mmol/L). Failure of regulation within this range results in altered concentrations of sodium and exposes cells to hypotonic (hyponatremia) or hypertonic (hypernatremia) stress.

HYPONATREMIA
Epidemiology

Hyponatremia (defined as a serum sodium <135 meq/L) is one of the most common electrolyte disorders encountered in clinical practice.[23,24] In the elderly population hyponatremia is especially common, and surveys of nursing home residents indicate a prevalence as high as 30%.[25]

Pathogenesis and diagnostic approach

Hypotonic hyponatremia, the most common form, results from impaired excretion of a dilute urine. In normal osmoregulation, thirst and vasopressin (antidiuretic hormone [ADH]) secretion are suppressed by dilute plasma sodium concentrations (<135 mmol/L). The presence of ADH is reflected by urine that is not maximally dilute (urine osmolality >100 mOsm/kg), indicating ongoing tubular water reabsorption. Baroreceptor activation in states of profound decrease in effective circulating volume (volume depletion, heart failure, cirrhosis) can stimulate ADH secretion despite the inhibitory effect of low serum sodium levels. In such cases, the kidney avidly reabsorbs sodium under control of aldosterone but rates of water reabsorption exceed sodium uptake, resulting in hyponatremia. ADH-mediated hyponatremia in the presence of normal perfusion and low serum osmolality may be considered "inappropriate." Simplified in the later section are common pathogeneses and causes of hyponatremia, with associated laboratory abnormalities. Diagnostic approach based on laboratory abnormalities is detailed in **Fig. 2**.

Hyponatremia with low urine osmolality (<100 mOsm/kg)

- Psychogenic polydipsia may lead water intake exceeding maximum capacity to excrete water. Chronic kidney disease may also be a risk factor for this development.

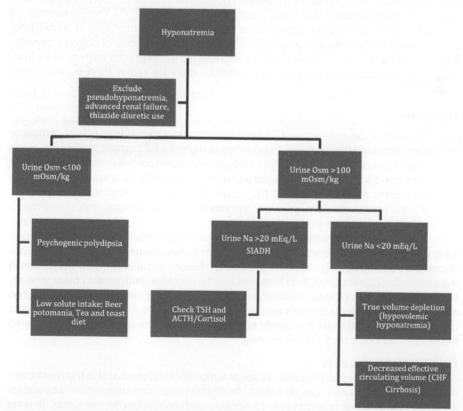

Fig. 2. Diagnostic approach to hyponatremia.

- Beer potomania or "tea and toast diet" (chronically low-solute intake inhibits water excretion).

Hyponatremia with intact antidiuretic hormone secretion (>100 mOsm/kg)

- True volume depletion most commonly seen in the ambulatory setting is caused by GI fluid losses (vomiting, diarrhea) and urinary losses (diuretic therapy, aldosterone deficiency), leading to activation of baroreceptors and ADH release with subsequent water retention.
- Hypervolemic hyponatremia in patients with heart failure or cirrhosis results from a low effective circulating arterial volume, which results in excessive thirst and ADH release. The degree of hyponatremia often correlates with severity of the disorder.
- Euvolemic hyponatremia—hyponatremic patients who are unable to dilute their urine in the absence of renal failure (impaired diluting ability) and thiazide use and are neither hypovolemic nor edematous are classified as having syndrome of inappropriate ADH (SIADH). SIADH is a diagnosis of exclusion and it is essential to determine its cause. Common causes are summarized in **Table 2**.

Complications

Mild chronic hyponatremia (plasma sodium concentration 125–135 mEq/L) is the most common electrolyte abnormality seen in the ambulatory setting. Clinical manifestations associated with untreated moderate hyponatremia include neurocognitive deficits, gait disturbances, fall risk, and bone fractures.[26–28] The presence of hyponatremia is associated with increased morbidity and mortality in ambulatory and hospitalized patients and is regarded as an important marker of disease severity. It is likely that the major mortality effect attributed to hyponatremia derives more from the underlying cause, leading to the electrolyte disorder rather than hyponatremia itself.[24,29,30]

Management

It is imperative to determine need for hospitalization in those at high risk of complications from untreated hyponatremia and those at high risk for complications from overcorrection of hyponatremia. Hospital management allows for frequent assessment of neurologic condition, accurate measurement of urine output, and water excretion as well as frequent measurements of the serum sodium concentration. Such patients include those with acute hyponatremia, symptomatic hyponatremia, and severe hyponatremia (sodium <120 mEq/L).

Correction of hyponatremia in the outpatient setting involves addressing the underlying cause. For patients with heart failure or cirrhosis, treatment with diuretics can improve serum sodium by improving renal perfusion. In patients with hypovolemic hyponatremia, correction of fluid loss and supplementation with either oral or isotonic IVFs will often correct the hyponatremia. In these instances though, patients will often self-correct with a water diuresis as volume status stabilizes.[31] Additional therapeutic options and their rationale are briefly summarized later. These strategies are geared mostly toward outpatient SIADH management.

Restriction of fluid intake

Restriction of fluid intake presents a logical option for treatment and is the most common first step taken by most clinicians. Its effectiveness can be predicted by examining the summed concentrations of sodium and potassium in the urine. If urine (Na + K) is less than half of serum sodium concentration, fluid restriction alone should

Table 2 Causes of syndrome of inappropriate antidiuretic hormone secretion	
Central nervous system disorders	Infarction, hemorrhage, vasculitis Brain surgery, trauma Neoplasm Infections Guillian-Barre syndrome
Pulmonary disorders	Pneumonia • Viral • Bacterial • Tuberculous Asthma
Malignancies	Small cell carcinoma of the lung Head and neck squamous cell tumors
Endocrine disorders	Glucocorticoid deficiency Severe hypothyroidism
Drugs (common causes)	Anticonvulsants • Carbamazepine • Sodium valproate • Lamotrigine Antipsychotics and antidepressants • Haloperidol • MAOIs • SSRIs • Tricyclic antidepressants • Venlafaxine Anticancer drugs • Vinca alkaloids • Platinum compounds • Cyclophosphamide • Methotrexate Nonsteroidal antiinflammatory drugs "Ecstasy"/MDMA
Others	Nausea Pain AIDS Alcohol withdrawal

Abbreviations: MAOIs, monoamine oxidase inhibitors; MDMA, methylenedioxymethamphetamine; SSRIs, selective serotonin uptake inhibitors.

result in gradual improvement of hyponatremia. (Recommended degrees of fluid restriction are detailed in expert recommendations, but generally 500 cc less than fluid loss[31]). If the urine cation concentration is greater than the serum sodium concentration (a concentrated urine), other measures in conjunction with fluid restriction are required (**Fig. 3**).

Promoting renal water excretion; increasing urine solute load and decreasing medullary concentration gradient

Currently, 2 strategies are used to increase urine solute load: enteral sodium chloride (NaCl) and urea. Sodium chloride is effective in hyponatremia partly by increasing urine solute load, causing an electrolyte diuresis. However, NaCl is usually used in conjunction with loop diuretics, primarily for prevention of negative sodium balance.[32] Usual doses for NaCl tablets are 6 to 9 g daily in 3 divided doses. Oral urea is another

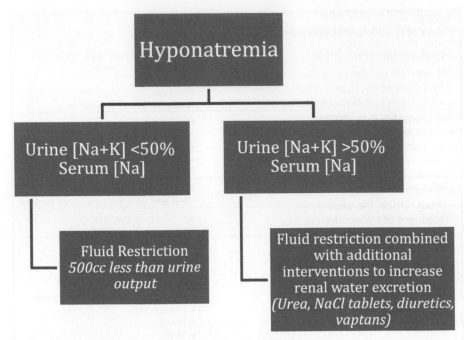

Fig. 3. Determining interventions for SIADH treatment.

option for management of outpatient hyponatremia by increasing water excretion by inducing an osmotic diuresis. It seems to be inexpensive and well tolerated in clinical trials.[33] The usual dose for maintenance therapy is 15 to 30 g/d.

Decreasing medullary osmotic gradient
Concurrent use of loop diuretics is beneficial in patients with high urine concentrations by impairing the formation of a concentrated urine in the collecting duct. Furosemide can be dosed up to 3 times daily and is effective in patients with SIADH, cirrhosis, and heart failure. In patients with SIADH, it may be used in combination with NaCl tablets.[34,35]

Inhibition of antidiuretic hormone actions in the kidney
Currently, there are 2 agents available that antagonize the renal action of ADH: demeclocycline and vasopressin receptor antagonists. Demeclocycline, although effective, is not approved by the Food and Drug Administration (FDA) for hyponatremia treatment, and the European guidelines on diagnosis and treatment of hyponatremia recommend against its use.[36] Vasopressin receptor antagonists (vaptans) produce a water diuresis, leading to correction in serum sodium. Currently, initiation of vaptan use requires inpatient management, with frequent monitoring of laboratories to avoid overcorrection. However, use is limited by cost, and the FDA recommends against its use for greater than 30 days.[37]

HYPERNATREMIA

Hypernatremia (defined as serum sodium >145 mEq/L) is much less common than hyponatremia, estimated to occur in 2% to 5% in acutely ill patients.[38,39] This is likely due to the individual's ability to obtain free water in the presence of an intact thirst mechanism. It is only when thirst is impaired (impaired cognition) or when water access limited that hypernatremia occurs.[40] When plasma sodium levels increase to greater than 145 mEq/L, high ADH levels produce maximally concentrated urine (~1200 mOsm/L). The presence of dilute urine in such circumstances implies deficient ADH secretion or failure of the kidneys to respond to ADH.

Most commonly, hypernatremia is caused by failure to replace fluid losses. Even in cases of complete diabetes insipidus, where urinary losses are electrolyte-free water, thirst is an effective defense preventing development of hypernatremia. Therefore, in the ambulatory setting, hypernatremia is seen most commonly in debilitated nursing home patients with deficient thirst mechanism and decreased access to water or may be unmasked following surgical procedures where general anesthesia precludes oral intake.[41,42] It can also be seen in infants where formula is incorrectly mixed. Rare case reports of exogenous sodium loading leading to symptomatic hypernatremia exist but remain the exception.[43]

Treatment of hypernatremia focuses on treating the underlying cause and repleting the free-water deficit. Because there is little effect on effective circulating blood volume, these patients typically will not necessitate resuscitative fluids but will need repletion of hypotonic fluid. The hypotonic fluid is preferably given as oral-free water or intravenous 5% dextrose in water if enteral access is not possible. Frequent monitoring of sodium should be done with a goal reduction of less than 12mEq/L Na in 24 hours.[42]

DISORDERS OF POTASSIUM BALANCE: HYPO- AND HYPERKALEMIA

Extracellular fluid and plasma potassium (K^+) concentrations are usually maintained in the 3.5 to 5.1 mEq/L range. Potassium is the dominant intracellular cation with 3000 to 3500 mmol located intracellularly and only 1% to 2% of total body potassium located in the extracellular fluid.[44] Normal cellular function requires potassium concentration within a narrow range, achieved by short-acting (transcellular shifts) and long-acting (renal and GI systems) regulatory systems.

HYPERKALEMIA

Kidney Disease: Improving Global Outcomes (KDIGO) recently defined acute hyperkalemia as "a potassium result above the upper limit of normal that is not known to be chronic." Generally, the potassium level is greater than 5.0 mEq/L but study definitions vary.[45] The potential causes of hyperkalemia are vast, with common ones listed in **Box 1**.

Epidemiology

Hyperkalemia is a rare finding in patients with normal renal function. Studies of renin-angiotensin system blocking agents including ACE inhibitors, angiotensin receptor blockers (ARBs), and aldosterone blockers suggest the incidence of hyperkalemia is less than 2% with a mean increase in serum potassium of 0.13 to 0.2 mEq/L.[46] In patients with chronic kidney disease (CKD), risk is stratified by GFR, with one study suggesting the incidence of serum potassium greater than 5.5 mEq/L at 3.1% in CKD stage 3 versus 13.7% in CKD stage 4.[47]

Evaluation

A new finding of hyperkalemia should prompt clinician investigation. Guidelines suggest an inpatient evaluation for a potassium level of greater than 6.0 mEq/L; however, for those with less severe hyperkalemia, a thorough search for medication and dietary causes should be undertaken. Patients with potassium level greater than or equal to 5.5mEq/L should have an electrocardiogram performed to evaluate for possible

> **Box 1**
> **Causes of hyperkalemia**
>
> - Artifactual findings such as pseudohyperkalemia from phlebotomy or tourniquet use
> - Transcellular shifts due to hyperosmolar states of cell lysis (rhabdomyolysis or tumor lysis syndrome)
> - Impaired distal nephron sodium delivery as may occur in decreased effective circulating volume
> - Inadequate GFR/reduced renal function to excrete a dietary potassium load
> - Hypoaldosteronism and low aldosterone-like states
> - Pharmacologic effects may occur from blockade of the renin-angiotensin-aldosterone system, NSAIDs, calcineurin inhibitor use, or potassium-sparing diuretics
>
> *Abbreviation:* NSAIDs, nonsteroidal antiinflammatory drugs.

conduction abnormalities. Pseudohyperkalemia can be confirmed ideally with a tourniquet-free repeated phlebotomy to confirm the diagnosis, and if possible, the blood sample should be processed on site to avoid cell lysis due to tube systems and courier transport.

Triage and Treatment of Hyperkalemia

As previously noted, recent KDIGO guidelines recommend inpatient evaluation of patients with potassium levels greater than 6.0 mEq/L and/or evidence of arrhythmia. A detailed discussion of inpatient management of severe, life-threatening hyperkalemia is beyond the scope of this review; however, outpatients can be successfully managed with mild to moderate hyperkalemia. A variety of strategies may be used including the following:

- Dietary potassium restriction[48]
  - Foods with high levels of potassium: dried fruits, molasses, avocados, nuts, bran cereal, lima beans, spinach, tomatoes, broccoli, carrots, potatoes, bananas, cantaloupe, oranges, mangos, red meat, pork, and lamb
- Enhanced renal excretion via diuretic usage
- GI sequestration of potassium via oral binding resins
- Withholding of causative medications such as ACE-Is, ARBs, or aldosterone blockers

Treatment should be tailored to the individual characteristics of the hyperkalemic patient with a balance of risks and benefits. For example, a patient with CKD may benefit from the kaliuretic effect of chlorthalidone while also reducing volume overload. However, a hyponatremic elderly patient may risk exacerbation of hyponatremia. Regarding diuretics, in general, thiazide diuretics lose efficacy with increased stages of CKD, and loops are preferred in stage 4 to 5 CKD.

Recently, 2 new potassium-binding resins received FDA approval—patiromer and zirconium cyclosilicate.[49,50] These are in addition to the existing sodium polystyrene sulfonate (SPS). Although all 3 are effective at lowering potassium, some consider SPS higher risk due to rare but persistent reports of bowel necrosis.[51] Neither patiromer nor zirconium cyclosilicate are approved for treatment of acute hyperkalemia but both effectively reduce chronic hyperkalemia. Medication withdrawal, such as ARB discontinuation in proteinuric kidney disease, must be balanced against the loss of renal protection these agents provide.

HYPOKALEMIA

A serum potassium concentration less than 3.5 mEq/L defines hypokalemia. A serum potassium concentration of 2.5 to 3 mEq/L is considered moderate and a level less than 2.5 mEq/L is regarded as severe hypokalemia.[52] Rates of hypokalemia have been shown to be 12% to 21% among hospitalized patients, largely of multifactorial cause with concomitant hypomagnesemia in most patients.[53,54]

Causes

Hypokalemia may result from 1 of 4 possible causes: pseudohypokalemia, redistribution between cellular compartments, GI losses, and renal losses. In addition, hypomagnesemia is strongly associated with hypokalemia and contributes to kidney losses. Common causes and clinical conditions associated with hypokalemia are listed in **Table 3**.[54]

Diagnostic Approach

The most common causes of hypokalemia in the ambulatory setting can be elucidated by the patient's clinical presentation. Differentiating urinary versus GI potassium loss can be elucidated by assessing urinary potassium excretion. Although a 24-hour urine potassium excretion is ideal, it may not always be feasible in the outpatient setting. Alternative useful measurements include the transtubular potassium gradient and the urine potassium to creatinine ratio. Both are estimates of urinary potassium handling, and a higher potassium excretion in hypokalemic patients indicates inappropriate renal potassium wasting. A urine potassium to creatinine ratio of less than 13 mEq/g creatinine indicates the hypokalemia is from GI losses, transcellular shifts, or poor intake.[55]

Clinical assessment of volume and blood pressure also provide additional clues to the state of mineralocorticoid excess or diuretic-like effect.

Management

Optimal correction of hypokalemia warrants a diagnosis of the cause and treatment of the underlying disorder. Symptoms from hypokalemia usually do not occur at serum potassium concentrations higher than 2.5 mEq/L. In addition to muscle weakness,

Table 3		
Causes and clinical conditions associated with hypokalemia		
Causes of Hypokalemia	**Clinical Conditions**	
Transcellular shifts; secondary to increased activity of the Na-K-ATPase pump	• Increased insulin availability (ie, refeeding syndrome) • Increased β-adrenergic activity • Thyrotoxicosis • Alkalosis • Hypokalemic periodic paralysis • Theophylline use	
Gastrointestinal losses (extrarenal losses)	• Vomiting • Diarrhea	
Renal losses	• Diuretic use (carbonic anhydrase inhibitors, thiazide, and loop diuretics) • Bartter/Gitelman syndromes • Primary aldosteronism • Liddle syndrome (apparent mineralocorticoid excess)	

severe potassium depletion can lead to muscle cramps, cardiac arrhythmias, and rhabdomyolysis.[56] In these cases, potassium chloride repletion in the hospital setting is recommended.

Mild to moderate hypokalemia (3–3.4 mEq/L) usually does not produce symptoms. Treatment can be initiated by oral potassium chloride, dose varying on the severity of hypokalemia. In patients with renal potassium wasting, a potassium sparing diuretic is often needed. In addition, hypomagnesemia increases distal potassium secretion. Magnesium levels should be checked and repleted in all cases of hypokalemia, as potassium supplementation is ineffective in the setting of hypomagnesemia.

SUMMARY

The maintenance of volume and electrolyte homeostasis is a critical function of the kidney. The primary care physician in the course of treating and monitoring chronic medical conditions and associated laboratories is very likely to encounter electrolyte abnormalities including sodium and potassium as well as fluid abnormalities.

The following are important considerations in managing electrolytes and volume balance:

- Use history, physical, and laboratory findings to guide volume assessment.
- Treatment of hypovolemia depends on the cause, but if patient can be managed as an outpatient either watered down juices/sports drinks or balanced oral rehydration therapy can be used.
- Hyponatremia is a common electrolyte abnormality with a multitude of causes, and treatment depends on cause.
  - For hypovolemic hyponatremia, correction of volume status with close monitoring of subsequent aquaresis is typically sufficient.
  - For hypervolemic hyponatremia, correction of cause of hypervolemia with diuretics is typically first line.
  - For euvolemic hyponatremia, specifically SIADH, after addressing underlying cause, fluid restriction of approximately 500 cc less than urine output is first-line treatment, with possible need for additional therapies (NaCl tablets, urea, vaptans, diuretics).
- Hypernatremia is less common and often due to lack of access to free water. Correction of no more than 12 mEq/L/d should be achieved through use of isotonic fluids, preferably enteric free water when access is available.
- Hyperkalemia often requires inpatient evaluation for values greater than 6.0 mEq/L; however, for milder asymptomatic cases outpatient management includes determining underlying cause.
  - Potassium binding resins
  - Diuretics (thiazide in normal or mildly depressed renal function, loop for CKD stage 4,5)
  - Withholding causative agent
- Hypokalemia can be caused by GI losses, transcellular shifts, or renal losses but is rarely symptomatic unless less than 2.5 mEq/L.
  - Management includes repletion with oral potassium chloride or use of potassium-sparing diuretics.
  - Hypomagnesemia must be corrected in hypokalemia for successful treatment

DISCLOSURE

The authors have nothing to disclose.

REFERENCES

1. Hoenig MP, Hladik GA. Overview of kidney structure and function. In: Bomback A, Perazella M, Tonelli M, editors. National kidney foundation. primer on kidney diseases. 7th edition. Philadelphia: Elsevier; 2018. p. 2–18.

2. Koeppen BM, Stanton BA. Physiology of body fluids. In: Renal physiology. 6th edition. Philadelphia: Elsevier; 2019. p. 1–13.

3. Bhave G, Neilsen E. Volume depletion vs dehydration: How understanding the difference can guide therapy. Am J Kidney Dis 2011;58(2):302–9.

4. Bailey MA, Unwin RJ. Renal Physiology. In: Feehally J, Floege J, Tonelli M, et al, editors. Comprehensive clinical nephrology. 6th edition. Elsevier; 2019. p. 14–28.

5. Bollag WB. Regulation of Aldosterone Synthesis and Secretion. In: Terjung R, editor. Comprehensive physiology;American physiology society: rockville, MD. 2014. p. 1017–55.

6. Narins RG, Krishna GC. Disorders of water balance. In: Stein JH, editor. Internal medicine. Boston: Little, Brown; 1987. p. 794.

7. Halterman R, Berl T. Therapy of dysnatremic disorders. In: Brady HR, Wilcox CS, editors. Therapy in nephrology and hypertension. Philadelphia: Saunders; 1999. p. 257–69.

8. Bowman BT, Rosner MH. Lixivaptan - an evidence-based review of its clinical potential in the treatment of hyponatremia. Core Evid 2013;8:47–56.

9. McGee S, Abernethy WB, Simel DL. Is this patient hypovolemic? JAMA 1999; 281(11):1022–9.

10. Johnson DR, Douglas D, Hauswald M, et al. Dehydration and orthostatic vital signs in women with hyperemesis gravidarum. Acad Emerg Med 1995;(2):692–7.

11. Mullangi S, Sozio SM, Segal P, et al. Point-of-care ultrasound education to improve care of dialysis patients. Semin Dial 2018;31(2):154–62.

12. Breidthardt T, Irfan A, Klima T, et al. Pathophysiology of lower extremity edema in acute heart failure revisited. Am J Med 2012;125(11):1124.e1-e8.

13. Agarwal R, Andersen MJ, Pratt JH. On the importance of pedal edema in hemodialysis patients. Clin J Am Soc Nephrol 2008;3(1):153–8.

14. Dossetor JB. Creatinemia vs Uremia. The relative significance of blood urea nitrogen and serum creatinine concentrations in azotemia. Ann Intern Med 1966; 65(6):1287–99.

15. Matsue Y, van der Meer P, Damman K, et al. Blood urea nitrogen-to-creatinine ratio in the general population and in patients with acute heart failure. Heart 2017; 103(6):407–13.

16. Blantz RC. Pathophysiology of pre-renal azotemia. Kidney Int 1998;53:512–23.

17. Diskin CJ, Stokes TJ, Dansby LM, et al. The comparative benefits of the fractional excretion of urea and sodium in various azotemic oliguric states. Nephron Clin Pract 2010;114(2):c145–50.

18. Carvounis CP, Nisar S, Guro-Razuman S. Significance of the fractional excretion of urea in the differential diagnosis of acute renal failure. Kidney Int 2002;62(6): 2223–9.

19. Chugh R, Beauvais J, Sanjana L, et al. Gastrointestinal bleed: A new look at an old trend. Am J Gastroenterol 2017;112(S1):S316.

20. Riddle M, DuPont H, Connor B. ACG clinical guideline: diagnosis, treatment and prevention of acute diarrheal infections in adults. Am J Gastroenterol 2016; 111(5):602–22.

21. Hew-Butler T, Rosner MH, Fowkes-Godek S, et al. Statement of the third international exercise-associated hyponatremia consensus development conference, Carlsbad, California, 2015. Clin J Sport Med 2015;25(4):303–20.
22. Convertino VA, Armstrong LE, Coyle EF, et al. American College of Sports Medicine position stand. Exercise and fluid replacement. Med Sci Sports Exerc 1996;28(1).
23. Upadhyay A, Jaber BL, Madias NE. Incidence and prevalence of hyponatremia. Am J Med 2006;119(7suppl1):S30–5.
24. Schrier RW, Sharma S, Shchekochikhin D. Hyponatremia: more than just a marker of disease severity? Nat Rev Nephrol 2013;9(1):37–50.
25. Cowen LE, Hodak SP, Verbalis JG. Age-associated abnormalities of water homeostasis. Endocrinol Metab Clin North Am 2013;42(2):346–70.
26. Gunathilake R, Oldmeadow C, McEvoy M, et al. Mild hyponatremia is associated with impaired cognition and falls in community-dwelling older persons. J Am Geriatr Soc 2013;61:1838–9.
27. Renneboog B, Musch W, Vandemergel X, et al. Mild chronic hyponatremia is associated with falls, unsteadiness, and attention deficits. Am J Med 2006;119:71.e1-e8.
28. Gankam Kengne F, Andres C, Sattar L, et al. Mild hypontramei and risk of fracture in the ambulatory elderly. QJM 2008;101:583–8.
29. Wald R, Jaber BL, Price LL, et al. Impact of hospital associated hyponatremia on selected outcomes. Arch Intern Med 2010;170(3):294–302.
30. Chawla A, Sterns RH, Nigwekar SU, et al. Mortality and serum sodium: do patients die from or with hyponatremia ? Clin J Am Soc Nephrol 2011;6(5):960–5.
31. Verbalis JG, Goldsmith SR, Greenberg A, et al. Diagnosis, evaluation and treatment of hyponatremia: expert panel recommendations. Am J Med 2013;126:S1–42.
32. Berl T. Impact of solute intake on urine flow and water excretion. J Am Soc Nephrol 2008;19:1076–8.
33. Rondon-Berrios H, Tandukar S, Mor MK, et al. Urea for treatment of hyponatremia. Clin J Am Soc Nephrol 2018;13(11):1627.
34. Mount DB. Thick ascending limb of the loop of Henle. Clin J Am Soc Nephrol 2014;9:1974–6.
35. Decaux G, Waterlot Y, Genette F, et al. Treatment of the syndrome of inappropriate secretion of antidiuretic hormone with furosemide. N Engl J Med 1981;304:329–30.
36. Spasovski G, Vanholder R, Allolio B, et al. Clinical practice guideline on diagnosis and treatment of hyponatraemia. Nephrol Dial Transplant 2014;29(Suppl 2):i1–39.
37. Schrier RQ, Gross P, Gheorghiade M, et al. SALT investigators: Tolvaptan, a selective oral vasopressin V2-receptor antagonist, for hyponatremia. N Engl J Med 2006;355:2099–112.
38. Arampatzis S, Frauchiger B, Fiedler GM, et al. Characteristics, symptoms and outcomes of severe dysnatremias present on hospital admission. Am J Med 2012;125(11):1125.e1–7.
39. Gucyetmez B, Ayyildiz AC, Ogan A, et al. Dysnatremia on intensive care unit admission is a stronger risk factor when associated with organ dysfunction. Minerva Anestesiol 2014;80(10):1096–104.
40. Shah MK, Workeneh B, Taffet GE. Hypernatremia in the geriatric population. Clin Interv Aging 2014;9:1987–92.
41. Bourque CW. Central mechanisms of osmosensation and systemic osmoregulation. Nat Rev Neurosci 2008;9:519–31.

42. Adrogue HJ, Madias NE. Hypernatremia. N Engl J Med 2000;342:1493–9.
43. Carlberg DJ, Borek HA, Syverud SA, et al. Survival of acute hypernatremia due to massive soy sauce ingestion. J Emerg Med 2013;45(2):228–31.
44. Weiner D, Linas SL, Wingo CD. Disorders of potassium metabolism. In: Feehally J, Floege J, Tonelli M, et al, editors. Comprehensive clinical nephrology. 6th edition. Elsevier; 2019. p. 111–23.
45. Clase CM, Carrero JJ, Ellison DH, et al. Potassium homeostasis and management of dyskalemia in kidney diseases: conclusions from a Kidney Disease: Improving Global Outcomes (KDIGO) Controversies Conference. Kidney Int 2020;97(1): 42–61.
46. Weir MR, Rolfe M. Potassium homeostasis and renin-angiotensin-aldosterone system inhibitors. Clin J Am Soc Nephrol 2010;5(3):531–48.
47. Maddirala S, Khan A, Vincent A, et al. Effect of angiotensin converting enzyme inhibitors and angiotensin receptor blockers on serum potassium levels and renal function in ambulatory outpatients: risk factors analysis. Am J Med Sci 2008; 336(4):330–5.
48. Gennari FJ. Hypokalemia. N Engl J Med 1998;339:451–8.
49. Bakris GL, Pitt B, Weir MR, et al. Effect of patiromer on serum potassium level in patients with hyperkalemia and diabetic kidney disease: the AMETHYST-DN Randomized Clinical Trial. JAMA 2015;314(2):151–61.
50. Packham DK, Rasmussen HS, Lavin PT, et al. Sodium zirconium cyclosilicate in hyperkalemia. N Engl J Med 2015;372(3):222–31.
51. McGowan CE, Saha S, Chu G, et al. Intestinal necrosis due to sodium polystyrene sulfonate (Kayexalate) in sorbitol. South Med J 2009;102(5):493–7.
52. Unwin RJ, Luft FC, Shirley DG. Pathophysiology and management of hypokalemia: a clinical perspective. Nat Rev Nephrol 2011;7:75–84.
53. Crop MJ, Hoorn EJ, Lindemans J, et al. Hypokalemia and subsequent hyperkalemia in hospitalized patients. Nephrol Dial Transplant 2007;22:3471–7.
54. Paice BJ, Paterson KR, Onyanga-Omara F, et al. Record linkage study of hypokalaemia in hospitalized patients. Postgrad Med J 1986;62:187–91.
55. Lin SH, Yin YF, Chen DT, et al. Laboratory tests to determine the cause of hypokalemia and paralysis. Arch Intern Med 2004;164:1561–6.
56. Rose BD, Post TW. Hypokalemia. In: Rose BD, Post TW, editors. Clinical physiology of acid-base and electrolyte disorders. 5th ediiton. New York: McGraw-Hill; 2001. p. 836.

Acute Kidney Injury

Jackcy Jacob, MD, FACP, FAAP[a],*, Joanne Dannenhoffer, MD, MS[b],
Annie Rutter, MD, MS[b]

KEYWORDS

- Acute kidney injury • Elevated creatinine • Kidney damage • Acute renal failure

KEY POINTS

- Acute kidney injury (AKI) is defined by changes in serum creatinine or changes in urine output over the course of hours to days.
- Because physical symptoms and even typical laboratory evidence of kidney injury are often not identified initially, early identification requires recognition of symptoms of the underlying cause.
- Severity of illness, suspected mechanism of renal insult, and availability of local resources dictate how and where the patient can be managed: in the ambulatory setting versus referral to an emergency room or nephrologist.
- Medications that can potentiate AKI or are renally excreted require cessation or dose adjustment as a critical step in AKI management.
- Management of AKI patients includes postevent screening of creatinine and urine output in addition to management of risk factors for recurrent AKI or development of chronic kidney disease.

INTRODUCTION

If the injury was followed by recovery, acute kidney injury (AKI) was once considered an isolated event. However, over the last several decades, it has become increasingly apparent that AKI is part of a broad clinical syndrome with important downstream consequences for the AKI survivors, including a tenfold higher risk of developing chronic kidney disease (CKD), and twofold increased risk of death compared with their counterparts without AKI.[1,2] It is also becoming more apparent that the setting in which the AKI has developed (eg, in the community, on the hospital ward, or in the intensive care unit [ICU]) has implications for the patient's prognosis and long-term care plan, as it often reflects the degree of morbidity and reversibility of renal dysfunction. In hospitalized patients, AKI increases length of stay in the hospital, cost of care, and mortality in the hospital.[2–4]

a Department of Medicine, Albany Medical College, 43 New Scotland Ave, Albany, NY 12208, USA; b Department of Family and Community Medicine, Albany Medical College, 43 New Scotland Ave, Albany, NY 12208, USA
* Corresponding author.
E-mail address: jacobj@amc.edu
Twitter: @jac2thersq (J.J.); @drjosiebif (J.D.); @AnnieRutterMD (A.R.)

Prim Care Clin Office Pract 47 (2020) 571–584
https://doi.org/10.1016/j.pop.2020.08.008
0095-4543/20/© 2020 Elsevier Inc. All rights reserved.
primarycare.theclinics.com

Primary care clinicians may need to initiate management when AKI is diagnosed in the ambulatory setting or follow-up the care of a patient with resolved AKI. Management is often based on the underlying cause of the AKI. Because most cases of AKI are managed by non-nephrologists, it becomes critical that generalists are acquainted with the risk factors, diagnosis, and acute and chronic management of these patients. There is currently minimal formal guidance on optimal management strategies for AKI, but data do suggest that these patients require closer follow-up than has previously been noted.[5]

DEFINITIONS

AKI has largely replaced the term acute renal failure as there can be injury, without complete failure of the renal system that can still result in adverse outcome. Thus, the broader terminology lends to considering kidney injury as a syndrome ranging from a small decrease in glomerular filtration rate (GFR) to complete loss of function requiring renal replacement therapy (RRT), which may help to identify at-risk individuals earlier (**Fig. 1**).[6]

Evolution of the Diagnosis

Increased consensus on definitions has led to a better understanding of the disease and increased epidemiologic data with everyone using consistent language. The first consensus definition of AKI was the 2004 RIFLE criteria (Risk, Injury, Failure, Loss, and End Stage Renal Disease), which was modified into the Acute Kidney Injury Network (AKIN) definition of 2007.[6,7] Those criteria were further refined in the 2012 Kidney Disease Improving Global Outcomes (KDIGO) Clinical Practice Guideline for Acute Kidney Injury. This is currently the most widely accepted definition of AKI and uses changes in serum creatine (SCr) and urine output (UOP) to create a staged model of AKI divided into 3 categories (**Fig. 2**).[8]

It should be noted, however, that this absolute criterion is less specific for AKI in patients with more advanced CKD, because a small rise in serum creatinine (SCr) in an individual with an elevated baseline creatinine may not represent a clinically important decline in GFR, whereas the same rise in an individual with a normal creatinine may indicate a marked decline in GFR.[9] The stage of AKI has been shown to correlate with both short- and long-term outcomes. The treatment is largely similar for most

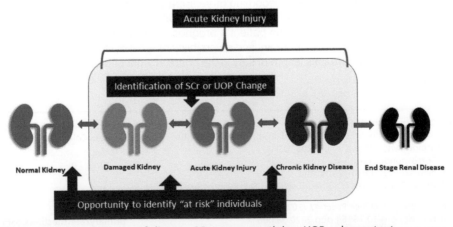

Fig. 1. AKI as a continuum of disease. SCr, serum creatinine; UOP, urine output.

Stage 1

Need only 1 criteria:

- [ ] SCr 1.5 to 1.9 times the baseline[a]
- [ ] >0.3mg/dL increase from the baseline
- [ ] Urine output <0.5mL/kg/h for 6–12 h

Stage 2

Need only 1 criteria:

- [ ] SCr 2.0 to 2.9 times the baseline
- [ ] Urine output <0.5mL/kg/h for >12 h

Stage 3

Need only 1 criteria:

- [ ] SCr 3 times the baseline
- [ ] SCr >4.0 mg/dL
- [ ] Starting RRT
- [ ] Urine output <0.5mL/kg/h for >24 h
- [ ] Anuria for >12 h

Fig. 2. Staging of AKI. RRT, renal replacement therapy; SCr, Serum Creatinine. [a] Baseline defined as lowest creatinine in the preceding 6 months. (*Data from* Kidney Disease Improving Global Outcomes Work Group. KDIGO clinical practice guideline for acute kidney injury. Kidney Int Suppl. 2012;2(1):1–138.)

of the stages, although with stage 2 and above, one may need to consider RRT or ICU admission (**Fig. 3**).[8]

Acute Kidney Disease

AKI and CKD are increasingly considered related entities and perhaps, a continuum of one disease state. Acute kidney disease (AKD) describes the patient with a subacute, ongoing pathophysiologic process between 7 to 90 days. It is used to describe the

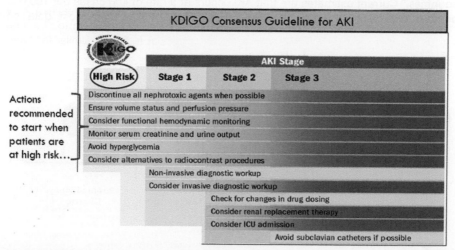

Fig. 3. Recognition of AKI and clinical responses. (*From* Acute Dialysis Quality Initiative 10. Available at http://www.adqi.org. ADQI *adapted from* Kidney Disease Improving Global Outcomes Work Group. KDIGO clinical practice guideline for acute kidney injury. Kidney Int Suppl. 2012;2(1):9; with permission.)

kidney that has suffered injury but is possibly on the mend and requires careful attention from clinicians. Research is ongoing as to the best ways to use this definition and ultimately how it will affect patients.[10]

Biomarkers

There has been considerable research over the last few decades of biomarkers that would act as adjuncts or earlier markers for the diagnosis of AKI. They would be used for risk assessment, determining underlying etiology, diagnosis and staging, prognosis, and management. Promising candidates include kidney injury molecule (KIM-1), cystatin-C, and neutrophil gelatinase-associated lipocalin (NGAL), among others but have yet to be incorporated into guidelines or integrated into routine clinical practice for the diagnosis or management of AKI.[11]

Community- and Hospital-Acquired Acute Kidney Injury

In an effort to better understand possible differences in risk factors and long-term prognosis, the incidence of AKI is commonly further characterized as community-acquired AKI (CA-AKI), which is present prior to admission to a hospital, and hospital-acquired AKI (HA-AKI), which develops during a hospital stay (**Fig. 4**). Of note, azotemia is a term that is often used incorrectly in place of AKI. Azotemia, defined as the biochemical increase in serum urea nitrogen (BUN), will result from severe reduction in kidney function and may be associated with oliguria or anuria, which is important to quantify when suspecting AKI, but is not synonymous with AKI.[12]

INCIDENCE/PREVALENCE

For decades, the reported incidence of AKI was noted to be variable based on differences in identifying, defining, and managing the disease, as well as variation in medical coding of the disease. Despite consensus in the definition based on the 2012 KDIGO guidelines, the numbers still seem dependent on the population studied. For example, there are more data in high-income countries than low- or middle-income countries.[6] Current estimates are that AKI occurs at a rate of 400 cases per 100,000 persons per year in community-based populations.[13] However, most data on

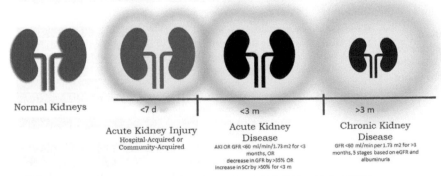

Fig. 4. General definitions. GFR, glomerular filtration rate; SCr, serum creatinine. (*Data from* Kidney Disease Improving Global Outcomes Work Group: KDIGO clinical practice guideline for acute kidney injury. *Kidney Int Suppl.* 2012;2(1):1–138.)

incidence are based on hospitalized patients, with some estimates that AKI affects up to 15% of hospitalized patients and 60% of ICU patients.[14] A patient database from the University of Pittsburgh suggests that about 33% of AKI cases are community acquired.[4] The incidence of AKI identified in community primary care offices is unclear.[3]

PATHOGENESIS/PATHOPHYSIOLOGY

AKI is often classified as prerenal, intrarenal (or intrinsic), and postrenal injury. Intrarenal represents true kidney injury with damage to 1 or more of the 4 major structures of the kidney: the tubules, the glomeruli, the interstitium, or the intrarenal blood vessels.[15] Pre- and postrenal injuries result from extrarenal diseases that lead to decreased GFR through impairment in autoregulation of renal blood flow and subsequent change to GFR. Normal GFR is determined by 2 factors: renal blood flow and the resistance in the afferent and efferent arterioles. The afferent arteriole dilates in the setting of low perfusion in order to maintain glomerular perfusion. If the renal compensatory mechanisms are already limited by certain comorbidities such as diabetes or concurrent medication use, or if the degree of reduced perfusion caused by the disease state cannot be overcome, renal injury develops.[16] Profound decreases in systemic vascular resistance (such as seen with splanchnic vasodilation in cirrhotic patients or in the form of septic or neurogenic shock) can also result in AKI, particularly when there is concurrent volume depletion or other insults.[17]

If the prerenal and postrenal conditions persist, it is possible for the damage to progress further and lead to intrinsic renal disease.[12] Although there are numerous potential causes of AKI, the pathophysiology is most often related to an impairment in the microcirculation, resulting in the mismatch between oxygen and nutrient delivery to the nephrons and increased energy demands (because of cellular stress), ultimately leading to inflammation, vascular injury, and tubular injury.[18] Of note, in CKD, renal afferent vasodilation is already functioning at maximal capacity in order to compensate for the reduced functional renal mass, thus maximizing GFR.[19] This impairment in autoregulation of renal blood flow is one of the main reasons why patients with underlying CKD are at a greater risk of AKI and prolonged complications after its occurrence.

CLINICAL AND LABORATORY PRESENTATION

Elevated SCr, relative to the patient's baseline, is the hallmark of AKI. Unknown preexisting CKD, however, may confound this diagnosis, as a chronically elevated SCr will make it challenging to distinguish AKI from CKD or AKI on CKD. There are some findings in the history and physical examination that may lend a clue; chronic conditions such as hypertension and diabetes may suggest CKD, especially in the absence of significant symptoms such as anasarca or change in urine color, which suggest a more acute process. Asymptomatic anemia may suggest a chronic process that is possibly related to underlying CKD. Common reasons for routine monitoring of SCr in the primary care setting include chronic conditions that can lead to CKD or the need for monitoring of medications, especially in patients at high risk for AKI (**Fig. 5**).

Although decreased urine output might be noted by the patient, an increase in serum creatinine level is typically not recognized clinically. Moreover, the symptoms from accumulation of nitrogenous wastes (eg, urea) are often nonspecific and delayed: confusion, lethargy, cramps, sleep disturbance, anorexia, nausea, amenorrhea, seizure, and even coma.[20] As such, the clinician must be adept at identifying features of the underlying cause of the AKI, be that poor renal perfusion or an obstructive kidney stone. The medication history should also be comprehensive enough to uncover

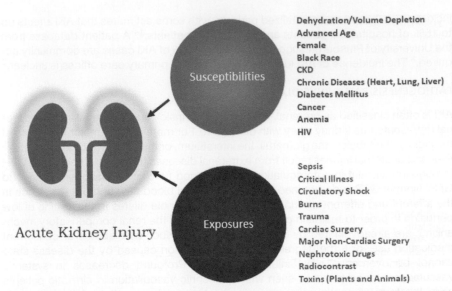

Susceptibilities

Dehydration/Volume Depletion
Advanced Age
Female
Black Race
CKD
Chronic Diseases (Heart, Lung, Liver)
Diabetes Mellitus
Cancer
Anemia
HIV

Acute Kidney Injury

Exposures

Sepsis
Critical Illness
Circulatory Shock
Burns
Trauma
Cardiac Surgery
Major Non-Cardiac Surgery
Nephrotoxic Drugs
Radiocontrast
Toxins (Plants and Animals)

Fig. 5. Exposures and susceptibilities for nonspecific AKI. CKD, chronic kidney disease; HIV, human immunodeficiency virus. (*Data from* Kidney Disease Improving Global Outcomes Work Group. KDIGO clinical practice guideline for acute kidney injury. Kidney Int Suppl. 2012;2(1):1–138.)

common nephrotoxic medications and medications that can potentiate renal injury in the presence of an additional insult (**Table 1**).

Prerenal

Prerenal AKI is caused by decreased blood perfusion of the kidneys, reduced renal blood flow, and thus, decreased GFR. Low flow states can be from volume depletion, such as from dehydration or hemorrhage, or from low effective circulating volume, such as with heart failure or liver disease with portal hypertension. The history is critical and can often lead to the underlying diagnosis even before the physical examination. Diarrhea, vomiting, or poor oral intake may suggest volume loss, especially when compounded by increased insensible losses such as from excessive sweating or persistent fevers. Signs of dehydration such as tachycardia, orthostatic hypotension, dry mucous membranes, skin tenting, or prolonged capillary refill may be present with dehydration or volume loss. A history of dyspnea on exertion along with abdominal ascites, lower extremity edema, or anasarca may be suggestive of hepatorenal or cardiorenal syndrome. In the hospitalized setting, the symptoms may be of other severe illnesses that can cause hypoperfusion, such as septic shock or major bleeding.[21]

Intrarenal

As with prerenal injury, the presenting symptoms of the diseases themselves and not the subsequent renal impairment may be the obvious diagnostic clue in intrinsic renal injury. For instance, the characteristic rash of systemic lupus erythematosus (SLE) or joint findings in rheumatologic disease may be the initial presenting signs of AKI. If a patient has fever and flank pain, this may be associated with pyelonephritis. Intrarenal AKI is typically caused by acute tubular necrosis (ATN) and is often precipitated by sepsis or an ischemic or toxic event. Thus, careful evaluation of drugs/medications and thorough examination for systemic infection become important.

Table 1
Medication management in acute kidney injury: commonly associated medications associated with acute tubular necrosis

Medications Commonly Associated with Acute Tubular Necrosis	Key Medications Requiring Dose Adjustment (or Cessation) in AKI
Aminoglycosides (tobramycin, gentamycin)	Analgesics (morphine, meperidine, gabapentin, pregabalin)
NSAIDs (ibuprofen, naproxen, ketorolac, celecoxib)	Antiepileptics (lamotrigine)
ACEi (captopril, lisinopril, benazepril, ramipril)	Antivirals
	Antifungals
ARB (losartan, valsartan, candesartan, irbesartan)	Antimicrobials
	Diabetic agents (sulfonylureas, metformin)
Amphotericin	Allopurinol
Cisplatin	Baclofen
Foscarnet	Colchicine
Iodinated contrast	Digoxin
Pentamidine	Lithium
Tenofovir	Low-molecular-weight heparin
Zolendronic acid	Direct Oral Anticoagulants

Adapted from Moore PK, Hsu RK, Liu KD. Management of acute kidney injury: core curriculum 2018. Am J Kidney Dis. 2018;72(1):139; with permission.

Postrenal

In postrenal obstruction, there is increased retrograde hydrostatic pressure with increased tubular pressure and ultimately, decreased GFR. Obstruction can occur at any level from the renal tubule to the urethra. Thus, history should focus on determining the underlying cause of the obstruction (ie, nephrolithiasis, prostatic disease, or pelvic or intra-abdominal mass). Again, symptoms are more likely related to that disease rather than the kidney injury itself: colicky abdominal pain, urinary retention, nocturia, abdominal or pelvic pain or fullness, or even hematuria, may indicate renal obstruction. For obstruction above the bladder to produce significant AKI, both kidneys would need to be involved (or 1 kidney in the case of a patient with a single functioning kidney). Alternatively, pre-existing CKD may develop into AKI with obstruction of only 1 kidney. Urinary obstruction may present as anuria or intermittent urine flow (such as polyuria alternating with oliguria) but may also present as nocturia, urinary incontinence, or purely nonoliguric AKI.[12]

INITIAL EVALUATION AND TREATMENT

Once AKI is diagnosed, initial evaluation should consider the need for urgent intervention and referral. Significant electrolyte abnormalities, stage 3 AKI, and the need for RRT are indications for immediate evaluation in the emergency department and early coordination of care with nephrologists. If those aforementioned situations are not present, the next step is to determine if the change is acute or chronic. Laboratory findings such as normocytic anemia or elevated phosphate levels are more suggestive of CKD rather than AKI.[21] Therefore, complete blood count and serum phosphorus level can be checked to aid in determination.

Identification and treatment of the underlying cause are paramount to initiating treatment, as any supportive care is secondary to reversal of the underlying condition.

As discussed previously, etiology of underlying conditions can be separated into 3 main diagnostic categories. These can often be differentiated using history and physical examination with some support from basic laboratory and radiologic testing.

Prerenal

If prerenal AKI is suspected (eg, as in the case of severe blood loss or reduced cardiac output [because of heart failure or liver disease]), checking serum electrolytes, urinalysis, and urinary diagnostic indices such as urine concentrations of sodium and creatinine may be useful, as they can be used to determine the BUN-to-creatinine ratio or to calculate fractional excretion of sodium or urea. A BUN-to-creatinine ratio of greater than 20:1 is often suggestive of prerenal cause of injury (**Table 2**).

Postrenal

Postrenal etiologies of renal failure stem from the inability of the renal collecting system to eliminate urine. The most common etiologies are benign prostatic hypertrophy, ureteral or urethral strictures, renal stones, or papillary necrosis. History and physical examination are, again, the mainstays of diagnosis but are significantly enhanced with appropriate imaging studies.

Table 2
Evaluation of the urine in AKI

Urine or Renal Indices	Suggested Diagnosis
Overall urinalysis - normal	Prerenal or postrenal
Urine protein: >1–2 g/d	Glomerular cause
Specific gravity: >1.020	Prerenal
Urine eosinophils	Allergic interstitial nephritis (ie, drug exposure)
Urinary sediment	
White cells/casts	Pyelonephritis, interstitial nephritis
Hyaline casts	Prerenal
Red blood cells	Glomerular, vascular, interstitial, or other structural (ie, stone, trauma)
Urinary sodium (mmol/L)	
>40	Intrinsic injury
<20	Prerenal
Urine osmolality (mOsm/kg H_2O)	
>500	Prerenal
<350	Intrinsic
Fractional excretion of sodium (%) 5 (urine Na x plasma Cr)/(plasma Na x urine Cr)	
<1	Prerenal
>2	Intrinsic renal
Fractional excretion of urea (%)	
<35	Pre-renal
>35	Intrinsic

Data from Kidney Disease Improving Global Outcomes. KDIGO clinical practice guideline for acute kidney injury: online appendices A–f. Available at: https://kdigo.org/wp-content/uploads/2016/10/KDIGO-AKI-Suppl-Appendices-A-F_March2012.pdf.

For example, in an older man with symptoms suggestive of obstruction, prostatic-specific antigen (PSA) level may be warranted.

Ultrasound is effective to diagnose hydronephrosis in the setting of obstructive uropathy, as it is over 90% sensitive for detection of urinary tract obstruction.[8] However, ultrasound alone may not reliably identify the exact site of obstruction, in which case further testing might be warranted. Treatment remains dependent on reversal of the underlying cause, so additional evaluation with other radiologic studies such as computed tomography (CT) without contrast may be indicated, as it better determines the level of obstruction. Findings of hydronephrosis caused by obstruction or persistent hematuria warrant urologic consultation for definitive treatment.

Intrarenal

Unlike prerenal or postrenal etiologies of kidney failure, intrarenal (or intrinsic renal) etiologies stem from damage to the renal tissue itself (**Table 3**). Based on the patient's history, specific serologic and hematologic testing can help with diagnosis. Examination of urine sediment and urine microscopy is often a mainstay of AKI evaluation, but can be variable in its utility in determining specific intrinsic renal causes (see **Table 2**). It is likely more useful in differentiating intrinsic renal from pre- or postrenal causes (eg, white blood cells on microscopy suggesting pyelonephritis) and is especially valuable in cases with suspected glomerulonephritis. Microscopic hematuria associated with deteriorating renal function or proteinuria should raise suspicion for acute glomerulonephritis. Urinary sediment may increase diagnostic confidence and may help to narrow the differential diagnosis; however, in skilled hands, specific analysis of urinary crystals can suggest specific etiologies such as tumor lysis syndrome or ethylene

Table 3 Causes of intrarenal acute kidney injury	
Intrarenal Causes of AKI	**Examples**
Vascular or microvascular	Renal artery stenosis TTP, HUS, APS, PHTN, cholesterol emboli, scleroderma, autoimmune Medications
Glomerular	Immune complex mediated (eg, SLE, idiopathic MPGN, postinfectious GN, endocarditis, immunoglobulin A nephropathy, HSP) or Pauci immune (eg, GPA, drug-induced)
Tubular	Medications Infection Hemolysis/rhabdomyolysis Ischemia
Interstitial	Medications (eg, antibiotics, PPI, NSAIDs) Infections (eg, pyelonephritis, *Legionella*) Immune-mediated (eg, Sjogren, SLE, sarcoid)

Abbreviations: APS, antiphospholipid antibody syndrome; GPA, granulomatosis with polyangiitis; HSP, Henoch-Schonlein Purpura; HUS, hemolytic uremic syndrome; MPGN, membranoproliferative glomerulonephritis; NSAIDs-nonsteroidal anti-inflammatory drugs; PHTN, pulmonary hypertension; PPI, proton pump inhibitor; SLE, systemic lupus erythematosus; TTP, thrombotic thrombocytopenic purpura.

Adapted from Moore PK, Hsu RK, Liu KD. Management of acute kidney injury: core curriculum 2018. Am J Kidney Dis. 2018;72(1):138; with permission.

glycol intoxication.[8] Prompt collaboration with nephrology in primary glomerular disease or rheumatology in autoimmune diseases can be helpful for diagnosis and treatment. Additionally, if initial evaluation does not reveal a definitive underlying cause, renal biopsy may be warranted (**Fig. 6**).

MANAGEMENT OF MEDICATIONS, FLUID BALANCE, ELECTROLYTE ABNORMALITIES

Although the primary goal in treating AKI is in treatment of the underlying cause, AKI can lead to several complications, and management is necessary for prevention of morbidity and mortality.

Medication Management

Management is twofold: first, elimination or avoidance of nephrotoxic agents, and second, dose adjustment of medications that are renally metabolized. Nephrotoxic agents (see **Table 1**) should be eliminated whenever possible, even if they are not the underlying cause of the AKI. These medications can often be cautiously restarted upon resolution of AKI depending on the concern for future recurrence. There are several drugs that can alter the ability of the kidney to maintain GFR, but the most common drugs are nonsteroidal anti-inflammatory drugs (NSAIDs), which inhibit renal prostaglandin production, thus, limiting renal afferent vasodilation and angiotensin converting enzyme inhibitors (ACEIs) and angiotensin receptor blockers (ARBs), which restrict renal efferent vasoconstriction. As such, these medications, in particular, become important to manage up front. Educating the patient that NSAIDS are harmful to the kidney and that contrast agents should be avoided may also be part of the short- or long-term management plan. Medications that

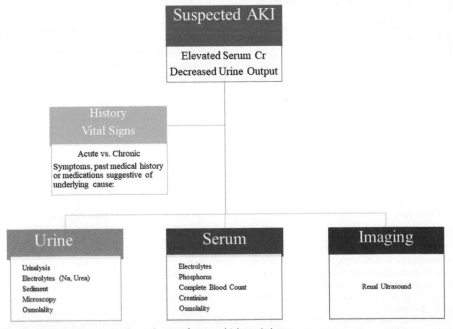

Fig. 6. Approach to initial work-up of acute kidney injury.

could lead to dehydration or reduction in renal blood flow, such as antihypertensives or diuretics, while not directly causing damage, may potentiate renal injury and should be stopped in many cases. However, there are some settings, such as in heart failure leading to AKI, where diuretics may in fact be indicated, as they help to manage fluid overload with accompanying ineffective circulation, and therefore can allow for recovery of the kidneys.[8]

When assessing which medications can accumulate in the setting of AKI, it is important to consider the patient's current renal function, and the anticipated trajectory of his or her recovery or progression. Equations that are typically used to estimate GFR such as Cockcroft-Gault, Modification of Diet in Renal Disease (MDRD), and CKD Epidemiology Collaboration (CKD-DPI) are not accurate when creatinine clearance is in flux, as during periods of AKI. The SCr measurement often lags behind the degree of injury or recovery. Therefore, one must be cautious when using it to determine actual GFR. Nevertheless, medication adjustments using creatinine clearance as a proxy for GFR are necessary. Kinetic estimations of GFR exist but are not commonly used. Although the Cockcroft-Gault equation is less accurate in patients at the extremes of body mass index (BMI) and age,[22] the MDRD equation was found to be less accurate in the setting of people without known kidney disease, so may be less helpful in the setting of AKI.[22] As most drug dosing suggestions are based on the Cockcroft-Gault equation, guidance from the National Kidney Disease Education Program suggests that either calculation can be used for drug dosing purposes.[23] Creatinine clearance should be recalculated periodically throughout treatment of AKI and dosing of medications likewise adjusted.

Fluids and Electrolytes

Other mainstays of treatment include management of the patient's volume status and electrolyte abnormalities. In prerenal AKI, intravenous fluid resuscitation is often necessary with attention to target blood pressure. Common serum and electrolyte abnormalities seen include hyperkalemia and metabolic acidosis. Although treatment and reversal of the underlying cause of AKI should address these electrolyte aberrations, sometimes, that process may be too slow. Acute attention to life-threatening metabolic disturbances requires urgent intervention and supersedes waiting for AKI resolution.

Nephrology Consultation/Referral Versus the Emergency Department

Location of treatment depends on the etiology and extent of kidney injury, as well as the resources available. Often, the underlying cause of AKI itself may be reason for hospitalization (such as in sepsis), but when the underlying etiologies can be treated and managed in the outpatient setting, anticipated success in restoring euvolemia and correcting electrolyte abnormalities safely dictate location of treatment.

Fluid resuscitation is often used in the treatment of AKI of various etiologies, but has been found to be helpful primarily in the setting of prerenal AKI and in contrast-induced nephropathy.[8] This can be done either orally or parenterally depending on the circumstances of the case. When considering RRT in the form of dialysis, indications for prompt referral include but are not limited to hyperkalemia, metabolic acidosis, symptoms or complications of uremia, fluid overload, and pulmonary edema.[24] In addition to RRT, indications for prompt nephrology referral include uncertainty about the cause of AKI, intrarenal etiology, inadequate response to treatment, stage 3 AKI, or in the setting of CKD.[24]

COMPLICATIONS AND PROGNOSIS

The natural course of AKI varies from complete renal recovery to dependency on dialysis or ultimately, death. AKI confers up to a tenfold higher risk of developing CKD and an increased risk of death compared to their counterparts without AKI.[1] Transient need for dialysis because of AKI with recovery of renal function placed patients at an especially high risk for progression to CKD, suggesting that the severity of the AKI is indeed a strong predictor of progression to CKD.[25] Additional risk factors for CKD after AKI include older age, a baseline GFR that was low to begin with, and albuminuria at baseline.[26] The severity of AKI at diagnosis can also affect the odds of death. In 1 study, as compared to patients without AKI, the risk of death in patients with KDIGO stage 1 AKI was 3.4 fold higher; stage 2 was 7.5 fold higher. Stage 3 was 13-fold higher, and those requiring dialysis had a 24-fold higher risk of death.[27] Interestingly, there is no difference between the long-term prognosis of patients with community-acquired AKI (CA-AKI) versus hospital-acquired AKI (HA-AKI) despite the higher prevalence of potentially more benign etiologies in CA-AKI compared with HA-AKI.[3] Both groups had worse outcomes than those without AKI; those with AKI had worse in-hospital mortality and longer length of stay as well as increased overall mortality. Patients with CA-AKI had more advanced stages of AKI than HA-AKI but did not need more acute RRT compared with HA-AKI.[28] A large study of hospitalized veterans with AKI found that 25% were ultimately rehospitalized within 1 year because of AKI. Most of those recurrences occurred within 3 months of discharge, suggesting another area of vigilance after the index AKI event.[5] AKI is also associated with an elevated risk of cardiovascular mortality and major cardiovascular events, particularly heart failure, acute myocardial infarction, and stroke.[29] Therefore, appropriate initial management and follow-up of patients with and recovering from AKI become important. Referral to a nephrologist is warranted in patients who do not recover renal function.

SUMMARY

Primary care providers are a powerful force in the initial management and transition from acute care of patients with AKI. The 2012 KDIGO guidelines suggest that a follow-up creatinine measurement is obtained within 3 months of resolution of AKI to monitor for early evidence of CKD or progression (ie, monitoring for proteinuria or reduced estimated glomerular filtration rate). Medication reconciliation, blood pressure control, and patient education are reasonable interventions until effective guidelines for AKI survivors are developed.[5] AKI is a common problem, but with early recognition and prompt management by the primary care provider in coordination with nephrologists, pharmacists, nursing, and laboratory personnel, the trajectory of the disease may in fact improve.

CLINICS CARE POINTS

- The diagnosis of AKI is made with a 1.5x (or higher) increase in creatinine or a decrease in urine output to <0.5 mL/Kg/hr.
- Significant electrolyte abnormalities, Stage 3 AKI, and the need for RRT are indications for immediate evaluation in the emergency department.
- Avoiding hyperglycemia, avoiding radioconstrast, and ensuring appropriate volume status are all important in safeguarding individuals at high risk for AKI.

ACKNOWLEDGMENTS

The authors thank Ms Elizabeth Irish and the Albany Medical College library for their contributions to this article. The authors also sincerely thank Dr Paul DerMesropian and Dr Loay Salman for their time and expertise in reviewing this content prior to publication.

DISCLOSURE

The authors have nothing to disclose.

REFERENCES

1. Coca SG, Singanamala S, Parikh CR. Chronic kidney disease after acute kidney injury: a systematic review and meta-analysis. Kidney Int 2012;81(5):442–8.
2. Chertow GM, Burdick E, Honour M, et al. Acute kidney injury, mortality, length of stay, and costs in hospitalized patients. J Am Soc Nephrol 2005;16(11):3365–70.
3. Wonnacott A, Meran S, Amphlett B, et al. Epidemiology and outcomes in community-acquired versus hospital-acquired AKI. Clin J Am Soc Nephrol 2014;9(6):1007–14.
4. Hackworth L, Wen X, Clermont GJ. Hospital versus community-acquired acute kidney injury in the critically ill: differences in epidemiology (abstr). J Am Soc Nephrol 2009;20:115A.
5. Silver SA, Siew ED. Follow-up Care in Acute Kidney Injury: Lost in Transition. Adv Chronic Kidney Dis 2017;24(4):246–52.
6. Mehta RL, Kellum JA, Shah SV, et al. Acute Kidney Injury Network: report of an initiative to improve outcomes in acute kidney injury. Crit Care 2007;11(2):R31.
7. Bellomo R, Ronco C, Kellum JA, et al. Acute renal failure - definition, outcome measures, animal models, fluid therapy and information technology needs: the Second International Consensus Conference of the Acute Dialysis Quality Initiative (ADQI) Group. Crit Care 2004;8(4):R204–12.
8. KDIGO Kidney Disease Improving Global Outcomes. Work Group. KDIGO clinical practice guideline for acute kidney injury. Kidney Int Suppl 2012;2(1):1–138.
9. Ostermann M, Joannidis M. Acute kidney injury 2016: diagnosis and diagnostic workup. Crit Care 2016;20(1):299.
10. Chawla LS, Bellomo R, Bihorac A, et al. Acute kidney disease and renal recovery: consensus report of the Acute Disease Quality Initiative (ADQI) 16 Workgroup. Nat Rev Nephrol 2017;13(4):241–57.
11. Coca SG, Yalavarthy R, Concato J, et al. Biomarkers for the diagnosis and risk stratification of acute kidney injury: a systematic review. Kidney Int 2008;73(9): 1008–16.
12. Makris K, Spanou L. Acute kidney injury: definition, pathophysiology and clinical phenotypes. Clin Biochem Rev 2016;37(2):85–98.
13. Hsu CY, McCulloch CE, Fan D, et al. Community-based incidence of acute renal failure. Kidney Int 2007;72(2):208–12.
14. Susantitaphong P, Cruz DN, Cerda J, et al. World incidence of AKI: a meta-analysis. Clin J Am Soc Nephrol 2013;8(9):1482–93.
15. Basile DP, Anderson MD, Sutton TA. Pathophysiology of acute kidney injury. Compr Physiol 2012;2(2):1303–53.
16. Burke M, Pabbidi MR, Farley J, et al. Molecular mechanisms of renal blood flow autoregulation. Curr Vasc Pharmacol 2014;12(6):845–58.
17. Bucsics T, Krones E. Renal dysfunction in cirrhosis: acute kidney injury and the hepatorenal syndrome. Gastroenterol Rep (Oxf) 2017;5(2):127–37.
18. Togel F, Westenfelder C. Recent advances in the understanding of acute kidney injury. F1000Prime Rep 2014;6:83.

19. Martens CR, Edwards DG. Peripheral vascular dysfunction in chronic kidney disease. Cardiol Res Pract 2011;2011:267257.
20. Meyer TW, Hostetter TH. Uremia. N Engl J Med 2007;357(13):1316–25.
21. Bellomo R, Kellum JA, Ronco C. Acute kidney injury. Lancet 2012;380(9843): 756–66.
22. Coresh J, Stevens LA. Kidney function estimating equations: where do we stand? Curr Opin Nephrol Hypertens 2006;15(3):276–84.
23. Stevens LA, Nolin TD, Richardson MM, et al. Comparison of drug dosing recommendations based on measured GFR and kidney function estimating equations. Am J Kidney Dis 2009;54(1):33–42.
24. Thomas, Mark, et al. National Clinical Guideline C. National Institute for Health and Clinical Excellence: guidance. In: Acute kidney injury: prevention, detection and management up to the point of renal replacement therapy. London: Royal College of Physicians (UK). National Clinical Guideline Centre; 2013. p. 164–9. Available at: https://www.ncbi.nlm.nih.gov/books/NBK247665/.
25. Chawla LS, Amdur RL, Amodeo S, et al. The severity of acute kidney injury predicts progression to chronic kidney disease. Kidney Int 2011;79(12):1361–9.
26. Schmitt R, Coca S, Kanbay M, et al. Recovery of kidney function after acute kidney injury in the elderly: a systematic review and meta-analysis. Am J Kidney Dis 2008;52(2):262–71.
27. Levey AS, James MT. Acute kidney injury. Ann Intern Med 2018;168(11):837.
28. Der Mesropian PJ, Kalamaras JS, Eisele G, et al. Long-term outcomes of community-acquired versus hospital-acquired acute kidney injury: a retrospective analysis. Clin Nephrol 2014;81(3):174–84.
29. Odutayo A, Wong CX, Farkouh M, et al. AKI and Long-Term Risk for Cardiovascular Events and Mortality. J Am Soc Nephrol 2017;28(1):377–87.

Chronic Kidney Disease

Cornelia Charles, MD[a], Allison H. Ferris, MD[b],*

KEYWORDS

- CKD • Chronic kidney disease • Chronic renal failure • Primary care • Albuminuria
- Slowing progression • Renal disease

KEY POINTS

- Chronic kidney disease is a common disease with increasing prevalence and is tied closely with diabetes and hypertension.
- The progression of chronic kidney disease can be slowed with several interventions including controlling blood pressure and diabetes.
- Both chronic kidney disease and the presence of albuminuria are risk factors for cardiovascular disease.
- Attention must be given to mitigating cardiovascular risk, avoiding drugs or interventions that can worsen renal function, and referring patients to a nephrologist when necessary.
- Primary care physicians play a key role in diagnosing and managing chronic kidney disease to slow its progression and prevent complications.

DEFINITION, EPIDEMIOLOGY, AND PREVALENCE

Kidney Disease: Improving Global Outcomes (KDIGO) in their 2012 Clinical Practice Guidelines for Evaluation and Management of Chronic Kidney Disease created a universal definition of chronic kidney disease that is widely applied to patient populations throughout the world.[1] Chronic kidney disease is defined as abnormalities of kidney structure or function, present for greater than 3 months with specific implications for health. This is defined as a GFR less than 60 mL/min/1.73 m^2 or one or more markers of kidney dysfunction including albuminuria. **Box 1** lists markers of kidney damage.

Chronic kidney disease is further classified into stages based on the estimated glomerular filtration rate (eGFR), as shown in **Table 1**.

According to the United States Renal Data System, it is estimated that 14.8% of the United States' general population was affected by chronic kidney disease in 2013 to 2016, with the most prevalent stage being chronic kidney disease stage 3.[2] The overall prevalence of chronic kidney disease in the United States has been stable for the last 2 decades, but when looking at stages, there has been a small increase in stage 3 from

[a] Department of Veterans Affairs Medical Center - West Palm Beach, 7305 North Military Trail, West Palm Beach, FL 33410; [b] Charles E. Schmidt College of Medicine, Florida Atlantic University, 800 Meadows Rd, Boca Raton, FL 33486
* Corresponding author.
E-mail address: ferrisa@health.fau.edu

Prim Care Clin Office Pract 47 (2020) 585–595
https://doi.org/10.1016/j.pop.2020.08.001
0095-4543/20/© 2020 Elsevier Inc. All rights reserved.

> **Box 1**
> **Criteria for chronic kidney disease (either of the following present for 3 months)**
>
> | | |
> |---|---|
> | Markers of kidney damage (≥1) | Albuminuria (albumin excretion rate ≥30 mg/24 h; albumin-to-creatinine ratio ≥30 mg/g [≥3 mg/mmol]) |
> | | Urine sediment abnormalities |
> | | Electrolyte and other abnormalities owing to tubular disorders |
> | | Abnormalities detected by histology |
> | | Structural abnormalities detected by imaging History of kidney transplantation |
> | Decreased GFR | GFR <60 mL/min/1.73 m^2 (GFR categories G3a–G5) |
>
> *Adapted from* Kidney Disease: Improving Global Outcomes (KDIGO) CKD Work Group. KDIGO 2012 clinical practice guideline for the evaluation and management of chronic kidney disease. Kidney Int Suppl. 2013;3:1–150; with permission. Copyright 2013.

2001 to 2016.[2] During that same time period, the prevalence of chronic kidney disease among patients with diabetes was around 36%, whereas it is 31% in individuals with hypertension.[2] Age has the highest correlation with low eGFR (eGFR <60 mL/min/1.73 m^2), and chronic kidney disease has the highest prevalence in individuals over the age of 60 years.[2,3] Compared with men, women have a slightly higher prevalence of both a GFR of less than 60 mL/min/1.73 m^2 (7.9% vs 6.4% per the above study) and albuminuria (10.9% vs 8.8%).[4]

The most common causes of chronic kidney disease in the United States are diabetes mellitus and hypertension, accounting for more than one-half of the cases. A higher body mass index (≥30 kg/m^2), cardiovascular disease, family history of kidney disease, black race, personal factors such as smoking or heavy alcohol use, medications, and other systemic diseases have also shown an association. Chronic kidney disease is an independent risk factor for cardiovascular disease, cognitive dysfunction, hospitalization, and all-cause mortality,[5] so its importance to primary care physicians cannot be understated.

Despite its prevalence, however, universal screening for chronic kidney disease in adults is not recommended; in fact, the US Preventative Services Task Force and

Table 1
GFR categories for chronic kidney disease

GFR Category	GFR (mL/min/1.73 m^2)	Terms
G1	≥90	Normal or high
G2	60–89	Mildly decreased
G3a	45–59	Mildly to moderately decreased
G3b	30–44	Moderately to severely decreased
G4	15–29	Severely decreased
G5	<15	Kidney Failure

Adapted from Kidney Disease: Improving Global Outcomes (KDIGO) CKD Work Group. KDIGO 2012 clinical practice guideline for the evaluation and management of chronic kidney disease. Kidney Int Suppl. 2013;3:1–150; with permission. Copyright 2013.

the American College of Physicians advises against screening asymptomatic individuals.[6,7] The American Society of Nephrology, however, recommends that those individuals at increased risk for chronic kidney disease should be screened, including those with diabetes, hypertension, or age above 55.[8]

PATHOGENESIS AND PATHOPHYSIOLOGY

Chronic kidney disease occurs as a consequence of 2 mechanisms: an initial trigger and a perpetuating mechanism.[9,10] The initiating stimulus can be a baseline kidney issue (it is abnormal from development or it is injured along the way), an inflammatory or immune-mediated cause, or a toxic insult. This kidney damage is then perpetuated by the process of hyperfiltration and hypertrophy of remaining nephrons. Several pathways can cause this: hormones (such as the renin–aldosterone system), cytokines, and growth factors. This process causes an increase in arterial filling pressure to the nephrons, thereby causing changes to the glomerular architecture and structure as well as changes to podocytes; this damages the filtration system. Ultimately, these continued insults lead to sclerosis of nephrons and a further decrease in renal function. Specific etiologies of chronic kidney disease are outlined elsewhere in this article, but a few entities and their mechanisms of action are discussed here with additional information of various specific diseases elsewhere in this issue.

Diabetes mellitus leads to chronic kidney disease by 3 main mechanisms.[11] First, hyperglycemia by itself causes increases in growth factor, angiotensin II, endothelin, and advanced glycation end products, all of which contribute to the hyperfiltration effect. Second, with hyperfiltration, the capillary pressure increases, which ultimately leads to changes in the glomerulus, including the classic thickened basement membrane, expanded mesangium, increase in extracellular matrix, and eventual fibrosis. As the kidney develops these changes, albuminuria develops, which is an additional risk factor for cardiovascular disease.[1]

Hypertensive changes to the kidney occur by a slightly different mechanism.[12] There is loss of the usual autoregulation of the afferent arteriole leading to hyperfiltration and, in response, the afferent arteriole undergoes vascular changes. As hyperfiltration persists, there is further damage and further worsening of hypertension, both at the systemic level and the glomerular level, perpetuating the cycle of insult and injury. Eventually glomerulosclerosis occurs and, finally, atrophy and/or necrosis.

Glomerulonephritides use another mechanism to initially injure the kidney and lead to chronic kidney disease.[13] It often starts with immune complexes depositing into the basement membrane, triggering the release of chemokines that draw in various neutrophils, T cells, and macrophages. These immune cells trigger a cascade of additional chemokines and cytokines that further perpetuate the inflammation and damage. Furthermore, there can be proteases, complements, and oxidants that directly damage the glomerular structure. Ultimately, interstitial nephritis develops, leading to loss of filtrating and concentrating abilities, causing proteinuria, which triggers more inflammatory mediators and activation of the renin–angiotensin system. This process then produces hypertensive and ischemic changes, and the damaged tubules trigger additional growth factors that eventually culminates in fibrosis and scarring.

Polycystic kidney disease is an example of a developmental kidney abnormality that leads to chronic kidney disease.[14] The development of cysts disrupts the architecture of the kidney and, as they grow, the cysts compress surrounding healthy tissue leading to obstruction and eventual death of healthy nephron units, triggering the ongoing decline of renal function. Additionally, this process releases cytokines, chemokines, and growth factors, which triggers inflammation and eventual fibrosis.

DIAGNOSIS

Chronic kidney disease is classified by cause, GFR category, and albuminuria category, also known as the CGA classification. Cause for chronic kidney disease is assigned based on presence or absence of systemic disease and the location within the kidney of observed or presumed pathologic–anatomic findings. Estimated risk of concurrent complications and future outcomes can be predicted by using GFR categories and level of albuminuria (**Fig. 1**).

Early stages of chronic kidney disease are typically asymptomatic, and symptoms do not manifest until stage G4 and G5 or when GFR falls below 30 mL/min/1.73 m^2. Metabolic abnormalities and electrolyte disturbances lead to complications, including anemia and secondary hyperparathyroidism.[4] Once chronic kidney disease has progressed to end-stage renal disease, several nonspecific symptoms can occur such as fatigue, nausea, loss of appetite, confusion, difficulty concentrating, irritability, insomnia, and pruritis. A careful history and physical examination can help to reveal the cause of the chronic kidney disease. Oftentimes, however, chronic kidney disease is incidentally found from serum chemistry panels that include a serum creatinine. The GFR should be estimated because this parameter provides a more accurate measure of renal function. This calculation can be accomplished by using creatinine-based equations that adjust for factors that affect serum creatinine and creatinine clearance including age, sex, race and muscle. Most widely used is the Chronic Kidney Disease Epidemiology Collaboration equation:[15]

$$GFR = 141 \times \min (Scr/x,1)^\alpha \times \max(Scr/x,1)^{-1.209} \times 0.993^{AGE} \times (1.018 \text{ if female}) \times (1.159 \text{ if black})$$

[Scr – serum creatinine, x – 0.7 for females and 0.9 for males, α – -0.329 for females and -0.411 for males, min – the minimum of Scr/x or 1, max – maximum of Scr/x or 1]

		Prognosis of CKD by GFR and Albuminuria Categories: KDIGO 2012		Persistent albuminuria categories Description and range		
				A1	**A2**	**A3**
				Normal to mildly increased	Moderately increased	Severely increased
				<30 mg/g <3 mg/mmol	30–300 mg/g 3–30 mg/mmol	>300 mg/g >30 mg/mmol
GFR categories (ml/min/ 1.73 m²) Description and range	G1	Normal or high	≥90			
	G2	Mildly decreased	60–89			
	G3a	Mildly to moderately decreased	45–59			
	G3b	Moderately to severely decreased	30–44			
	G4	Severely decreased	15–29			
	G5	Kidney failure	<15			

Green: low risk (if no other markers of kidney disease, no CKD); Yellow: moderately increased risk; Orange: high risk; Red, very high risk.

Fig. 1. Prognosis of chronic kidney disease by GFR and albuminuria categories. (*Adapted from* Kidney Disease: Improving Global Outcomes (KDIGO) CKD Work Group. KDIGO 2012 clinical practice guideline for the evaluation and management of chronic kidney disease. Kidney Int Suppl. 2013;3:1–150; with permission. Copyright 2013.)

The Modification of Diet in Renal Disease equation similarly can be used in estimating GFR, but this equation is less accurate for a GFR of greater than 60 mL/min/1.73 m^2. Additionally, certain conditions that affect the GFR, such as extremes of muscle mass or diet, may require the measurement of cystatin C, and the GFR can be confirmed using the Chronic Kidney Disease Epidemiology creatinine–cystatin equation.[16] In assessing for albuminuria, the primary care physician should order a random urine albumin–creatinine ratio.

Further laboratory testing should include serum electrolytes (sodium, potassium, chloride, and bicarbonate), urinalysis (for specific gravity, pH, red blood cells, and leukocyte counts), and complete blood count.[17,18] Because chronic kidney disease is an independent risk factor for cardiovascular disease, a lipid panel should also be obtained. A renal ultrasound examination should be ordered in all patients with chronic kidney disease to look for hydronephrosis, cysts, or stones and to assess the size, symmetry, and echogenicity of the kidneys.[17] If suggested by the history, antinuclear antibodies can be obtained to evaluate for lupus, serologic testing for hepatitis B and C as well as human immunodeficiency virus, serum antineutrophil cytoplasmic antibodies to evaluate for vasculitis, and serum and urine protein immunoelectrophoresis for multiple myeloma.[17] If the prior evaluation is not indicative of the etiology of the chronic kidney disease, a kidney biopsy should be considered to determine etiologies that are less common, including unexplained tubulointerstitial disease, glomerulonephritis, or membranous nephropathies (**Table 2**).

MANAGEMENT

The management of chronic kidney disease revolves around slowing the progression of the disease and minimizing additional insults to the kidney. The primary care physician has an important role in this process given that they are likely the first person to recognize the decline in GFR and best know the patient's comorbidities and contributing factors for worsening chronic kidney disease. Predictors of progression are listed in **Table 3**.[19]

Although some of the predictors are modifiable, others such as age and sex are obviously not. The "other" category includes predictors that may be partially modified, but not fully, because the damage has already been done. In any event, the primary care physician should work with the patient to control those factors that are able to be modified. Resources such as the 2012 KDIGO guidelines are a great source of information for primary care physicians to help guide the care of these patients. Ultimately, there are 4 interventions that are shown to delay progression of chronic

Table 2		
Suggested initial studies for patients with suspected chronic kidney disease		
All Patients	**If Suggested by History**	**If Etiology Still Not Clear**
Basic metabolic panel	Antinuclear antibodies	Renal biopsy
Urinalysis	Hepatitis B and hepatitis C serology	–
Complete blood counts	Human immunodeficiency virus	–
Lipid profile	Antineutrophil cytoplasmic antibodies	–
Renal ultrasound examination	SPEP, UPEP	–

Abbreviations: SPEP, serum protein electrophoresis; UPEP, urine protein electrophoresis.

Table 3		
Predictors of progression in chronic kidney disease		
Modifiable	**Nonmodifiable**	**Other**
Hypertension	Age	Cause of chronic kidney disease
Hyperglycemia	Sex	GFR level
Dyslipidemia	Race/ethnicity	Amount of albuminuria
Smoking	–	Presence of cardiovascular disease
Obesity	–	–
Use of nephrotoxic agents	–	–

kidney disease: controlling hypertension, using renin–angiotensin–aldosterone system blockers, managing diabetes and hyperglycemia, and correcting metabolic acidosis.[20]

Managing Comorbidities

Hypertension is one of the most important comorbidities to control in patients who have chronic kidney disease, regardless of whether it was hypertension that initially lead to the chronic kidney disease or not. Both the JNC8 and the KDIGO guidelines (1B recommendation) recommend keeping blood pressure less than 140/90 mm Hg in patients who have chronic kidney disease.[19,21] If a patient already has albuminuria, there is some evidence (2D recommendation) to support keeping the blood pressure at less than 130/80 mm Hg to help slow the progression of chronic kidney disease, with an additional suggestion to use an angiotensin-converting enzyme inhibitor or angiotensin receptor blocker if the albuminuria is greater than 300 mg/24 h.[19]

Because it is well-known that hyperglycemia ultimately damages the kidney and diabetes is a leading cause of chronic kidney disease in the United States, it is critical to control blood sugars. KDIGO gives a 1A recommendation to keep the hemoglobin A1c around 7%, with the permission to be more liberal if the patient has a limited life expectancy.[19] Patients with chronic kidney disease are at risk of hypoglycemia owing to decreased metabolism of the medications used to treat diabetes, so any patient who has already had issues with hypoglycemia can also be allowed to have a higher A1c if needed.

Given the high rate of cardiovascular disease in patients with chronic kidney disease, special attention must be given to screening for and treating this entity. KDIGO gives a 2B recommendation to putting patients with chronic kidney disease on low-dose aspirin unless there is an increased bleeding risk.[19] Most patients with chronic kidney disease should also be considered for statin therapy given their increased risk of cardiovascular disease.[19,20]

Lifestyle recommendations cannot be overlooked in patients with chronic kidney disease. The KDIGO guidelines give a 1C recommendation to limiting sodium to less than 2000 mg/d. Additionally, they give level 2 evidence to limiting protein intake to less than 0.8 g/kg/d in both diabetic and nondiabetic patients with G4 to G5 chronic kidney disease. Primary care physicians should strongly consider referring patients to nutritionists familiar with chronic kidney disease (1B recommendation) because they can often assist patients in making good food and beverage choices, taking into consideration protein, calories, micronutrients, and electrolytes. Furthermore, patients should be encouraged to do 150 min/wk of aerobic exercise, keep their body mass index between 20 and 25, and not smoke tobacco products (all 1D recommendations).[19]

Managing Sequelae of Chronic Kidney Disease

Anemia

Anemia is a common complication of chronic kidney disease. Given that 80% of the body's erythropoietin comes from the kidney's peritubular interstitial cells, it is no surprise that erythropoietin production decreases as the GFR decreases.[22] As the GFR decreases to less than 60, annual measurement of hemoglobin is suggested.[9] As the hemoglobin decreases to less than 10 g/dL, erythropoietin treatment is given, usually subcutaneously (because this route allows lower doses to be used than if given intravenously) with a goal hematocrit of 33% to 35% within 2 to 4 months.[22] Special attention should be paid to iron stores as well, often providing supplemental iron if the ferritin is less than 100 or the transferrin saturation is less than 20%.

Calcium, phosphorus, parathyroid hormone, and bones

The complex interplay of calcium, phosphorus, and parathyroid hormone on bone health necessitates monitoring in patients with chronic kidney disease. KDIGO gives a 1C recommendation to measuring and monitoring calcium, phosphorus, parathyroid hormone, and alkaline phosphatase when the GFR decreases to less than 45.[19] Primary care physicians should aim to maintain phosphorus levels in the normal range (2C recommendation) by suggesting a decreased dietary intake of phosphorus and using phosphate binders with meals to limit their absorption. Physicians should also aim to manage the secondary hyperparathyroidism by using agents such as calcitriol, paricalcitol, or cinacalcet,[23] but generally this would be done by a nephrologist, because secondary hyperparathyroidism as a consequence of chronic kidney disease is an indication for referral to nephrology.[19,20] Although patients with chronic kidney disease are at risk of bone disease, it is not recommended (2B evidence) to routinely test the bone mineral density in these patients.[19]

Metabolic acidosis

Serum bicarbonate levels are an important factor to monitor in patients with chronic kidney disease. KDIGO recommends (2B) to keep the serum bicarbonate in the normal range, supplementing when the level is <22 mmol/L. Oral supplement options include sodium bicarb 650 mg 3 times per day or sodium citrate 30 mL/d.[20]

Protecting the Kidney from Nephrotoxins

The kidney is a major system for drug metabolism and excretion; therefore, it is important to consider the effect of any medication or agent on the kidneys when it is prescribed. Some drugs require dose adjustment, whereas others should be avoided entirely. Sometimes it is not feasible to avoid a drug that is potentially nephrotoxic; therefore, it is important to closely monitor renal function during and after treatment with such an agent. Some over-the-counter medications and supplements have unknown effects on the kidney and in chronic kidney disease; therefore, herbal supplements should not be used, and any over-the-counter medications should be discussed with a physician or pharmacist before using (1B recommendation).[19]

Contrast agents present a special dilemma for primary care physicians, especially when patients may need radiologic studies to diagnose other medical conditions. Like with many situations in medicine, the risks and benefits must be considered before ordering any diagnostic test that requires the use of contrast agents. In regards to iodinated radio contrast agents, KDIGO recommends avoiding high-osmolar agents (1B recommendation), use the lowest dose (no grade), hold any other potentially nephrotoxic drugs periprocedurally (1C recommendation), allow adequate hydration before, during, and after the procedure (1A recommendation), and measure the GFR 2 to 3 days after the test (1C recommendation).[19] Gadolinium-based contrast should be avoided in patients with a GFR less than 15 (1B recommendation), and it is suggested to use a special formulation of gadolinium in patients whose GFR is less than 30 (2B recommendation).[19]

Vaccines

The immune system in patients with chronic kidney disease is impaired, raising their risk of infection. For this reason, KDIGO recommends vaccinating against influenza

Table 4
Summary of recommendations for managing patients with chronic kidney disease

Recommendation	Who	Grade of rec/ Level of Evidence
BP <140/90 mm Hg	All	1B
BP <130/80 mm Hg	Chronic kidney disease with albuminuria	2D
ACE-I/ARB treatment	Albuminuria >300 mg/24 h	1B
A1c ~7% (can be more liberal if short life expectancy or high risk of hypoglycemia)	All patients with DM	1A
Dietary sodium <2000 mg/d	All	1C
Dietary protein <0.8 g/kg/d	G4-5	2C if patient with DM, 2B if patient without DM
Referral to nutritionist	All	1B
Exercise >150 min/wk	All	1D
Goal body mass index 20–25	All	1D
No smoking	All	1D
Check Hgb annually; anemia if <13 (male), <12 (female)	All	No grade
Keep serum bicarbonate normal	All	2B
Check calcium, phosphorus, parathyroid hormone, and alkaline phosphatase	GFR of <45	1C
Daily low-dose aspirin	All who are at risk of chronic kidney disease (and not at high risk of bleeding)	2B
Vaccines		
Influenza		1B
Pneumococcal		1B
Hepatitis B (if likely to need RRT)	All	1B

Abbreviations: A1c, glycosylated hemoglobin; ACE-I, angiotensin-converting enzyme inhibitor; ARB, angiotensin receptor blocker; BP, blood pressure; DM, diabetes mellitus; Hgb, hemoglobin; RRT, renal replacement therapy.

Box 2
When to refer to a nephrologist

GFR less than 30 mL/min/1.73 m^2

Greater than 25% decrease in GFR

Progression of chronic kidney disease (sustained decline of GFR >5 mL/min/1.73 m^2 per year)

Significant albuminuria

Unexplained hematuria that is persistent

Complications of chronic kidney disease: secondary hyperparathyroidism, worsening anion gap acidosis, non–iron deficiency anemia

chronic kidney disease with hypertension requiring ≥4 medications

Persistent hyperkalemia or hypokalemia

Nephrolithiasis that is recurrent or extensive

Hereditary etiology of chronic kidney disease

Unknown etiology of chronic kidney disease

Data from Inker LA, Astor BC, Fox CH, et al. KDOQI US commentary on the 2012 KDIGO clinical practice guideline for the evaluation and management of CKD. Am J Kidney Dis. 2014;63(5):713–35.

(1B recommendation) and pneumococcal (1B recommendation) disease. Additionally, for patients who have advanced chronic kidney disease and are expected to progress to needing renal replacement therapy, it is suggested to vaccinate against hepatitis B (1B recommendation) (**Table 4**).[19]

NEPHROLOGY CONSULTATION AND REFERRAL

Although primary care physicians can mitigate further damage to kidneys and decline in renal function, there are specific instances in which referral to a nephrologist is recommended.[1,19] Given the chance of requiring renal replacement therapy in the near future, any patient with a GFR of less than 30 mL/min/1.73 m^2 should be managed by a nephrologist. Having that relationship early allows for proper discussions and planning for future needs in regards to possible dialysis or transplant consideration. Additionally, any patient with a 25% or greater decrease in the GFR or progressive worsening of the GFR of more than 5 mL/min/1.73 m^2 per year should also be referred to nephrology for further evaluation and management. Significant albuminuria (albumin/creatinine ratio of >300 mg/g or albumin excretion rate of ≥300 mg/24 h) is also an indication to consult a nephrologist, unless the etiology is known to be diabetes and the primary care physician is appropriately managing both the diabetes and the albuminuria. **Box 2** lists reasons to consider a nephrology referral in patients with chronic kidney disease.

SUMMARY

Chronic kidney disease is an entity that all primary care physicians need to be comfortable diagnosing and managing. Although diabetes and hypertension are the most common etiologies of chronic kidney disease, understanding the pathophysiology and comorbid conditions associated with chronic kidney disease will help the primary care physician to better assess and manage these patients. Attention must be given to mitigating cardiovascular risk, avoiding drugs or interventions that can worsen renal function, and referring patients to a nephrologist when necessary.

DISCLOSURE

The authors have nothing to disclose.

REFERENCES

1. Kidney Disease: Improving Global Outcomes (KDIGO) CKD Work Group. KDIGO 2012 clinical practice guideline for the evaluation and management of chronic kidney disease. Kidney Int Suppl 2013;3:1–150.
2. United States Renal Data System. 2018 USRDS annual data report: epidemiology of kidney disease in the United States. Bethesda (MD): National Institutes of Health, National Institute of Diabetes and Digestive and Kidney Diseases; 2018. Available at: https://www.usrds.org/2018/download/v1_c01_GenPop_18_usrds.pdf. Accessed January 12, 2020.
3. Murphy D, McCulloch CE, Lin F, et al. Centers for Disease Control and Prevention Chronic Kidney Disease Surveillance Team. Trends in prevalence of chronic kidney disease in the United States. Ann Intern Med 2016;165:473–81.
4. CDC: Centers for Disease Control and Prevention. National Health and Nutrition Examination Survey (NHANES). Available at: http://www.cdc.gov/nchs/nhanes.htm. Accessed January 12, 2020.
5. Levey AS, deJong PE, Coresh J, et al. The definition, classification, and prognosis of chronic kidney disease: a KDIOGO Controversies Conference Report. Kidney Int 2011;80:17–28.
6. U.S. Preventive Services Task Force Issues Final Recommendation Statement for Screening for Chronic Kidney Disease. U.S. Preventive Services Task Force. 2012. Available at: https://www.uspreventiveservicestaskforce.org/Announcements/News/Item/us-preventive-services-task-force-issues-final-recommendation-statement-for-screening-for-chronic-kidney-disease. Accessed January 12, 2020.
7. Saunders MR, Cifu A, Vela M. Screening for chronic kidney disease. JAMA 2015; 314:615–6.
8. Berns JS. Routine Screening for CKD Should Be Done in Asymptomatic Adults … Selectively. Clin J Am Soc Nephrol 2014;9:1988–92.
9. Bargman JM, Skorecki KL. Chronic kidney disease. In: Jameson J, Fauci AS, Kasper DL, et al, editors. Harrison's principles of internal medicine, 20e. New York: McGraw-Hill. Available at: http://accessmedicine.mhmedical.com.ezproxy.fau.edu/content.aspx?bookid=2129&sectionid=186950702. Accessed January 14, 2020.
10. Perlman RL, Heung M. Renal disease. In: Hammer GD, McPhee SJ, editors. Pathophysiology of disease: an introduction to clinical medicine, 8e. New York: McGraw-Hill. Available at: http://accessmedicine.mhmedical.com.ezproxy.fau.edu/content.aspx?bookid=2468&sectionid=198223240. Accessed January 10, 2020.
11. Powers AC, Stafford JM, Rickels MR. Diabetes mellitus: complications. In: Jameson J, Fauci AS, Kasper DL, et al. editors. Harrison's Principles of Internal Medicine, 20e New York: McGraw-Hill. Available at: http://accessmedicine.mhmedical.com.ezproxy.fau.edu/content.aspx?bookid=2129&sectionid=192288577. Accessed January 14, 2020.

12. Kotchen TA. Hypertensive vascular disease. In: Jameson J, Fauci AS, Kasper DL, et al, editors. Harrison's principles of internal medicine, 20e. New York,: McGraw-Hill. Available at: http://accessmedicine.mhmedical.com.ezproxy.fau.edu/content.aspx?bookid=2129&sectionid=192030227. Accessed January 14, 2020.

13. Lewis JB, Neilson EG. Glomerular diseases. In: Jameson J, Fauci AS, Kasper DL, et al, editors. Harrison's principles of internal medicine, 20e. New York: McGraw-Hill. Available at: http://accessmedicine.mhmedical.com.ezproxy.fau.edu/content.aspx?bookid=2129&sectionid=192281295. Accessed January 14, 2020.

14. Bergmann C, Guay-Woodford LM, Harris PC, et al. Polycystic kidney disease. Nat Rev Dis Primers 2019;4(1):50.

15. Matsushita K, Mahmoodi BK, Woodward M, et al. Chronic Kidney Disease Prognosis Consortium. Comparison of risk-prediction using the CKD-EPI equation and the MDRD study equation for the estimated glomerular filtration rate. JAMA 2012;307:1941–52.

16. Inker LA, Schmid CH, Tighiouart H, et al, CKD-EPI Investigators. Estimating glomerular filtration rate from serum creatinine and cystatin C. N Engl J Med 2012;367:20–9.

17. Drawz P, Rahman M. In the clinic: chronic kidney disease. Ann Intern Med 2015;162(11):ITC1.

18. Improving Global Outcomes (KDIGO) Anemia Work Group. KDIGO Clinical Practice Guideline for Anemia in Chronic Kidney Disease. Kidney Int Suppl 2012;2:279–335.

19. Inker LA, Astor BC, Fox CH, et al. KDOQI US Commentary on the 2012 KDIGO Clinical Practice Guideline for the Evaluation and Management of CKD. Am J Kidney Dis 2014;63(5):713–35.

20. Vassalotti JA, Centor R, Turner BJ, et al. Practical Approach to Detection and Management of Chronic Kidney Disease for the Primary Care Physician. Am J Med 2016;129:153–62.

21. James PA, Oparil S, Carter BL, et al. 2014 Evidence-based guideline for the management of high blood pressure in adults: report from the panel members appointed to the Eighth Joint National Committee (JNC 8). JAMA 2014;311(5):507–20.

22. Kaushansky K, Kipps TJ. Hematopoietic agents: growth factors, minerals, and vitamins. In: Brunton LL, Hilal-Dandan R, Knollmann BC, editors. Goodman & Gilman's: the pharmacological basis of therapeutics, 13e. New York: McGraw-Hill; Available at: http://accessmedicine.mhmedical.com.ezproxy.fau.edu/content.aspx?bookid=2189&sectionid=172481461. Accessed January 12, 2020.

23. Hypercalcemia and hypocalcemia. In: Jameson J, Fauci AS, Kasper DL, et al. eds. Harrison's manual of medicine, 20th ed. New York: McGraw-Hill; Available at: http://accessmedicine.mhmedical.com.ezproxy.fau.edu/content.aspx?bookid=2738&sectionid=227559880. Accessed January 14, 2020.

Nephrotic Syndrome

Seth Anthony Politano, DO[a],*, Gates B. Colbert, MD[b],
Nida Hamiduzzaman, MD[a]

KEYWORDS

- Nephrotic • Proteinuria • Dyslipidemia • Thrombotic • Membranous • Lupus
- Edema • Focal segmental glomerulosclerosis

KEY POINTS

- Glomerular disease is one of the major causes of end-stage kidney disease in the United States; prompt evaluation cause should be pursued to prevent further damage.
- Nephrotic syndrome commonly presents as edema, hypoalbuminemia, hypertension, dyslipidemia, and the presence of nephrotic-range proteinuria.
- Careful attention should be paid to the serious complications of nephrotic syndrome, including thrombotic events and infections.
- An investigation into the cause of nephrotic syndrome should be initiated as soon as possible, and a cost-effective and guided workup for secondary causes should be pursued.
- Treatment of the nephrotic syndromes generally includes sodium restriction, blood pressure control, management of edema, and treatment of dyslipidemia and complications. Therapy for the specific cause is initiated in conjunction with subspecialist consultation.

INCIDENCE AND PREVALENCE

Glomerular disease, including nephrotic syndrome and nephritic syndrome, is the third leading cause of end-stage kidney disease (ESKD) in the United States after diabetes mellitus and hypertension. Nephrotic syndrome predominantly affects men more than women.[1] In North America, the most common causes of nephrotic syndrome are diabetic nephropathy, focal segmental glomerulosclerosis (FSGS), and membranous nephropathy.

Diabetes mellitus is the leading cause of chronic kidney disease (CKD) and ESKD worldwide. In many countries, including the United States, diabetes is responsible for more than 40% of new cases of ESKD.[2] Besides causing nephropathy, diabetes can lead to irreversible complications such as diabetic retinopathy, diabetic neuropathy, and peripheral vascular disease.

[a] Division of GHPGIM, Keck School of Medicine of USC, 2020 Zonal Avenue, IRD 306, Los Angeles, CA 90089, USA; [b] Texas A&M College of Medicine, 3417 Gaston Avenue, Suite 875, Dallas, TX 75246, USA
* Corresponding author. 210 North Hudson Avenue, Apartment 2402, Pasadena, CA 91101.
E-mail address: politano@med.usc.edu

Prim Care Clin Office Pract 47 (2020) 597–613
https://doi.org/10.1016/j.pop.2020.08.002
0095-4543/20/© 2020 Elsevier Inc. All rights reserved.

The prevalence of FSGS seems to be increasing worldwide and is a major contributor to ESKD.[3] FSGS is the most common form of nephrotic syndrome in African American patients. A population-based study in the southwestern United States examined 2501 adult kidney biopsies performed between the years 2000 and 2011. Over the 12 years studied, FSGS was the most common diagnosis (39% of biopsies), with an increasing incidence rate from 1.6 to 5.3 patients per million[3,4]

Membranous nephropathy is the leading cause of nephrotic syndrome in Caucasian adults. In the United States, the incidence of membranous nephropathy is estimated at about 12 per million per year with a mean age between 50 and 60 and a 2:1 male predominance. The incidence of ESKD owing to membranous nephropathy in the United States is about 1.9/million per year. Because only 10% to 20% of patients with primary membranous nephropathy currently progress to ESKD, the real incidence may be as high as 20 per million per year.[5] Approximately 75% of cases are considered primary; the remaining 25% are typically secondary to diseases such as systemic lupus erythematosus, hepatitis B virus infection, solid tumors, and syphilis, as well as medications such as pencillamine and captopril. The diagnostic value of serum M-type phospholipase A2 receptor (PLA2R) antibody expression in patients with primary membranous nephropathy has been established. The M-type PLA2R is the specific podocyte antigen responsible for eliciting immune complex formation with circulating autoantibodies. Anti-PLA2R antibodies are detected in approximately 75% of primary cases and are rarely found in secondary forms. Also, patients with positive serum M-type PLA2R antibody area have a worse clinical remission rate; those with a higher titer of serum M-type PLA2R antibody have a lower chance of clinical remission and a higher risk of kidney failure without affecting relapse.[6]

Various demographic trends of glomerular disease in Southeastern United States have been studied. Overall, the frequency of membranous nephropathy declined significantly over the study interval, whereas, the incidence of diabetic nephropathy increased significantly. The frequency of FSGS increased initially, but it plateaued and ultimately declined.[6,7]

Minimal change disease (MCD) is the most common cause of the nephrotic syndrome in children (>90% of cases in children >1 year of age). In adults, MCD is the cause in 10% to 15% of cases of nephrotic syndrome, with a greater representation in older patients.[8]

PATHOGENESIS AND PATHOPHYSIOLOGY

Damage or dysfunction to the components of the glomerulus, including the basement membrane, the endothelial surface, or epithelial cells (podocytes), leads to loss of proteins (predominantly albumin) in the urine. Owing to limitations of the pore size in the basement membrane, as well as the charges of the barriers involved, only certain proteins can be lost through the urine.[9]

Owing to loss of albumin in the urine, oncotic pressure decreases, thereby decreasing circulating volume. This volume change is sensed by the juxtaglomerular apparatus and stimulates the renin–angiotensin axis leading to sodium and fluid retention. Patients with nephrotic syndrome have an inability to excrete sodium in the distal nephron, leading to volume retention and hypertension.[10]

The distinct pathophysiologic mechanism behind the causes of nephrotic syndrome varies widely by disease state. Antibodies that target the PLA2-r on podocytes are the most likely causes of primary membranous nephropathy and is thus considered a renal-specific autoimmune disease.[11] T-cell and B-cell activation likely play a role in MCD. FSGS can result from circulating factors and podocyte mutations.[12]

The hypercoagulable state encountered with nephrotic syndrome has multifactorial causes. The loss of proteins with similar masses to that of albumin occur in the syndrome, including protein S and antithrombin. In addition, fibrinogen and factors V and VIII are elevated.[12,13] There are also data supporting that the fibrin clot formation is altered in patients with nephrotic syndrome.[14] A prothrombotic state may also occur as fluid is leaked from the glomerulus, because it is currently not known all factors that are lost in the urine filtrate.[14,15] Nonetheless, the balance of increased procoagulant and loss of anticoagulants seems to be the driving force toward hypercoagulability. There is also evidence that hyperlipidemia seen in nephrotic syndrome promotes thrombosis via platelet activity.[16]

The mechanism for dyslipidemia in the nephrotic syndrome is complex and occurs through a variety of mechanisms. Patients often have a loss of lipoprotein lipase activators, malfunctioning anchors, and decreased hepatic lipase activity. Overall, this process leads to increased production of low-density lipoprotein cholesterol and decreased breakdown of low-density lipoprotein cholesterol and triglycerides. There is also overexpression of proprotein convertase subtilisin/kexin type 9, resulting in more low-density lipoprotein cholesterol remaining in the circulation. These altered lipids not only increase the risk of cardiovascular complications, but also can deteriorate renal function.[16]

CLINICAL AND LABORATORY PRESENTATION

By definition, the nephrotic syndrome is characterized by the loss of 3.0 to 3.5 g of protein in the urine in a 24-hour period, or a spot urine protein/creatinine value of 3.0 to 3.5 mg. Routine urinalysis can be performed the screen for proteinuria, although this method testing has shortcomings and can poorly predict the presence of proteinuria in the nephrotic range.

The most common presenting symptom of nephrotic syndrome is edema, particularly in the lower extremities. As the disease advances, or at times with initial presentation, patients can develop edema involving the sacrum, genitalia, abdomen, and proximal lower extremity. Anasarca can occur as well. Other findings owing to low oncotic pressure that can occur on presentation include pleural effusions and periorbital edema, although the latter is less likely in adults. Generalized fatigue and exertional dyspnea may be present even in early stages of the disease. Low albumin can cause Muehrcke lines (narrow white transverse lines) on the nails (**Fig. 1**).

Patients with nephrotic syndrome are likely to have hypertension at some point during their disease. In addition, the loss of immunoglobulins in the urine can predispose patients to infections, as well as local changes in the skin owing to edema. Various infections can occur, but cellulitis is the most common owing to this barrier disruption caused by edema.

Because patients with the nephrotic syndrome are hypercoagulable, an initial presentation may be of a venous thrombotic event (VTE). Arterial thrombosis is a less common but potential complication. The incidence of VTE during the course of disease in adults varies widely, but approximately one-third of patients will nephrotic syndrome will experience a VTE.[15] The most common site of thrombosis is in the lower extremities. Sometimes VTE can be asymptomatic, such as the case of incidentally found pulmonary embolism.[17] Patients can present with renal vein thrombosis (RVT) in the setting of previously undiagnosed nephrotic syndrome. Even though the risk of thrombosis increases with age overall, the acute presentation of RVT is more likely in younger patients, and can be accompanied by hematuria. Older patients are more

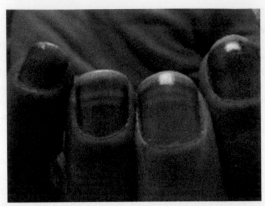

Fig. 1. Muehrcke lines. (*From* Tosti A. Diseases of hair and nails. In: Goldman L, Schafer Al, editors. Goldman-Cecil medicine. 26th edition, volume 2. Philadelphia: Elsevier; 2020. p. 2661; with permission.)

likely to have chronic presentations of RVT with chronic pain. Bilateral RVT, although rare, can present with acute kidney injury.[13,15]

Additional laboratory changes in nephrotic syndrome are closely related to the pathophysiology of the disease. Patients can present with hypoalbuminemia, and levels of less than 2.5 g/dL are likely to be found. Hyperlipidemia can also be found on laboratory tests, with elevated total cholesterol and triglyceride levels.[16] high-density lipoprotein cholesterol levels are usually unchanged.[18] Kidney function in many cases of nephrotic syndrome is progressive in nature, and markers of kidney function including the blood urea nitrogen and creatinine are usually within normal in most cases at initial presentation. As progression of the disease occurs however, CKD can develop with rising levels of these laboratory values.

In addition to the aforementioned findings in patients with nephrotic syndrome, the clinical presentation can vary depending on the cause of glomerular injury (**Table 1**).

DIAGNOSIS OF NEPHROTIC SYNDROME

Nephrotic syndrome can have primary or secondary etiologies as mentioned elsewhere in this article. Primary causes of nephrotic syndrome are MCD, primary and secondary membranous nephropathy, and FSGS. Secondary causes of nephrotic syndrome are diabetes mellitus, lupus nephritis, amyloidosis, and multiple myeloma. Of note, IgA nephropathy and membranoproliferative glomerulonephritis can also present as nephrotic syndrome, but with a nephritic component as well.

Nephrotic syndrome should be suspected in patients with edema, hypoalbuminemia (albumin <2.5 g/dL) and urine protein-creatinine ratio of greater than 3.0 to 3.5 mg. All patients with nephrotic syndrome should have a serologic workup to investigate causes (**Box 1**). A kidney biopsy is needed in some cases for a definitive diagnosis.

- Primary causes
    MCD
        MCD is the most common nephrotic syndrome in children; therefore, the diagnosis is based on the clinical picture. A kidney biopsy is not performed unless patients do not respond to glucocorticoid therapy. In adults, MCD has been associated with nonsteroidal anti-inflammatory drug use,

Table 1
Causes of nephrotic syndrome with associated clinical features

Secondary Cause	Clinical Presentation	Laboratory Presentation
Diabetes mellitus	Polyuria, polydipsia, polyphagia (usually earlier than nephrotic syndrome develops), fatigue, neuropathy, retinopathy, peripheral vascular disease	Elevated glucose, HgbA1c (note these can normalize as GFR declines)
Systemic lupus erythematosus	Arthritis, malar rash, discoid rash, photosensitivity, oral ulcers, serositis (pleuritic/pericardial/abdominal), neurologic dysfunction (depression, psychosis, stroke)	Elevated inflammatory markers, leukopenia, anemia, thrombocytopenia, renal dysfunction, elevated PTT, positive ANA, double-stranded DNA antibody, Smith Antibodies
Sjögren syndrome	Dry eyes, dry mouth, parotitis, arthritis, peripheral neuropathy, cough	Positive ANA, SSA/SSB
Cryoglobulinemia	Palpable purpura, acrocyanosis, livedo reticularis, arthritis, peripheral neuropathy	Elevated globulin fraction, monoclonal gammopathy, abnormal κ light chain/λ light chain ratio. Positive rheumatoid factor. Can have findings of nephritic syndrome (dysmorphic red blood cells/red blood cell casts in urine)
Amyloidosis	Orthostasis, peripheral neuropathy, diarrhea, heart failure, conduction abnormalities (ie, heart block), macroglossia, hypopigmented macular rash, pinch purpura (AL amyloidosis), hepatomegaly. If AA amyloidosis, examination may reveal findings consistent with primary disease (ie, rheumatoid arthritis)	Elevated alkaline phosphatase, findings consistent with primary cause (ie, myeloma, chronic inflammatory disorders)
Carcinoma	Varies depending on primary	Varies depending on primary
Hematologic malignancy (multiple myeloma, leukemia, lymphoma)	Myeloma—lytic lesions, symptoms of anemia, symptoms of hypercalcemia Leukemia—infections,	Hypercalcemia, renal failure, anemia, abnormal blood smear, thrombocytopenia, peripheral neuropathy

(continued on next page)

Table 1
(continued)

Secondary Cause	Clinical Presentation	Laboratory Presentation
	symptoms of anemia, bleeding	
Syphilis	Depending on stage—chancre, lymphadenopathy, fever, aortitis, gummas, altered mental statis, posterior column disease	Positive RPR/VDRL and FTA-ABS
Human immunodeficiency virus	Fatigue, lymphadenopathy, rash, opportunistic infections	Leukopenia, anemia, thrombocytopenia
Hepatitis B and C	May have findings consistent with liver disease (icterus, splenomegaly, caput medusa, ascites, palmar erythema, testicular atrophy)	Low platelets, elevated PT/INR, Any combination of abnormal liver function tests including ALP, AST, ALT, bilirubin elevations

Abbreviations: ALP, alkaline phosphatase; ALT, alanine aminotransferase; ANA, antinuclear antibody; AST, aspartate aminotransferase; FTA-ABS, fluorescent treponemal antibody absorption test; HgbA1c, hemoglobin A1c; GFR, glomerular filtration rate; PTT, partial thromboplastin time; RPR/VDRL, rapid plasma reagin/Venereal Disease Research Laboratory; SSA/SSB, Sjogren's Syndrome A/Sjogren's Syndrome B.

Box 1
Recommended serologic workup for Nephrotic Syndrome

- Urinalysis with microscopy
- Spot urine protein:creatinine ratio
- Complete blood count
- Comprehensive metabolic panel
- Hemoglobin A1C
- Complement panel
- Hepatitis panel
- Human immunodeficiency virus
- Antinuclear antibody with titer
- Serum protein electrophoresis and urine protein electrophoresis
- Serum free light chains
- PLA2R

Hodgkin's lymphoma, and lithium use. MCD is diagnosed with kidney biopsy demonstrating normal glomerular histology on light microscopy, negative immunofluorescence staining for immunoglobulin and complement proteins, and complete effacement of the podocyte foot processes on electron microscopy.

Membranous nephropathy

The diagnosis of membranous nephropathy is made by kidney biopsy, which shows the presence of spikes in the glomerular basement membrane on light microscopy using a Jones stain. The spikes are actually subepithelial peaks around the unstained immune deposits in the glomerular capillary wall, which are seen clearly on electron microscopy. Testing for serum PLA2R antibody is necessary, although the biopsy should also be stained for the PLA2R antigen, which has a higher sensitivity (>80%) than antibody testing in the serum alone. This serology helps to distinguish primary from secondary forms of the disease, especially because secondary forms can recur.[5] Because solid tumors are a risk factor, it is important to also screen all patients with an age-appropriate malignancy workup once this diagnosis is established. Other etiologies of membranous nephropathy include nonsteroidal anti-inflammatory drug use, autoimmune diseases (predominantly lupus), syphilis, and hepatitis B and C; therefore, testing for these diseases is necessary as clinically indicated. There are many more uncommon causes of secondary membranous nephropathy (including many autoimmune and inflammatory conditions such as sarcoidosis and Hashimoto's disease) and should be investigated when suspected given the clinical history.

FSGS

FSGS is common in African Americans owing to the APOL1 gene variation.[5,19] FSGS can also occur in patients with long standing hypertension, human immunodeficiency virus, obesity, hepatitis C, and heroin use. Like all nephrotic syndromes, FSGS is diagnosed by kidney biopsy. On light microscopy, glomerulosclerosis (scarring of glomeruli) is seen in a focal (<50%) and segmental (affecting a portion but not the entirety of individual glomeruli) distribution. Primary and secondary forms are usually differentiated by podocyte effacement quantification under electron microscopy.

- Secondary causes

Diabetic nephropathy

The diagnosis of diabetic nephropathy should be considered in patients with long-standing diabetes, proteinuria, and evidence of microvascular complications (nephropathy, neuropathy, or retinopathy) or macrovascular complications (stroke, ischemic heart disease, or peripheral arterial disease). A biopsy is usually only indicated for definitive diagnosis if the presentation is not consistent with diabetic nephropathy. On light microscopy, Kimmelstiel Wilson or nodular sclerosis are pathognomonic for diabetic nephropathy. Please see the Ryan Bonner and colleagues' article, "Diabetic Kidney Disease," in this publication on diabetic nephropathy for more information regarding the renal manifestations of diabetes mellitus.

Lupus nephritis

Lupus nephritis can present as nephritis or nephrosis. Nephritis will have a dysmorphic red blood cell or red blood cell casts, elevated serum creatinine, edema, and proteinuria. Nephrosis can present with these findings with nephrotic range proteinuria or can present with only nephrotic range proteinuria. A positive anti–double-stranded DNA antibody is necessary along with low complements. A kidney biopsy is important to determine the stage (**Table 2**) of lupus nephritis for diagnosis and management. A kidney biopsy is also indicated in a patient with established lupus nephritis with an unexplained increase in creatinine, active sediment, proteinuria of greater than 1 g/24 hours, or hematuria with proteinuria of 500 mg/24 hours.[20,21]

Amyloidosis

Amyloidosis kidney disease usually causes nephrotic range proteinuria and is most commonly caused by AL amyloid (primary) or AA amyloid (secondary). AL amyloid is composed of monoclonal κ or λ light chains. AA amyloid is produced by amyloid A protein and most commonly seen in chronic inflammatory diseases such as rheumatoid arthritis, inflammatory bowel disease, and chronic osteomyelitis. Therefore, in patients with kidney failure, if the ratio of serum free light chains is greater than 3, then the diagnosis of amyloidosis is likely. Tissue biopsy is needed to confirm the diagnosis; the sensitivity of abdominal fat pad aspiration is around 85%, rectal biopsy is 75% to 85%, and bone marrow biopsy about 50%.[20] Biopsy classically shows apple green birefringence under polarized light using a Congo red stain.

Multiple myeloma

Multiple myeloma should be considered in patients with calcium levels of greater than 11 mg/dL, serum creatinine of more than 2 mg/dL, hemoglobin of less than 10 g/dL, and lytic bone lesions. The presence of monoclonal light chains and an M protein spike is significant for multiple myeloma. Bone marrow biopsy usually shows greater than 10% clonal plasma cells or evidence of bony or extramedullary plasmacytoma. Kidney biopsy is only indicated if myeloma kidneys cannot be differentiated from other etiologies such as diabetic nephropathy. See **Table 3** for an overview of these causes.

MANAGEMENT OF NEPHROTIC SYNDROME

Once a diagnosis of nephrotic syndrome has been established, it is then important to treat with the intention to cure. Treating the disease that is causing glomerular damage

Table 2
Classification of lupus nephritis with biopsy findings

Classification	Biopsy Findings
Class I: minimal mesangial	No light microscopy abnormalities
Class II: mesangial proliferative	Mesangial hypercellularity or matrix expansion
Class III: focal	<50% of glomeruli have endocapillary and or extracapillary proliferation or sclerosis
Class IV: diffuse	>50% of glomeruli have endocapillary and or extracapillary proliferation or sclerosis
Class V: membranous	Diffuse thickening of the glomerular capillary walls with subepithelial deposits
Class VI: advanced sclerosing	>90% of glomeruli are globally sclerosed

Table 3
Summary of etiologies of nephrotic syndrome

	Demographics	Pathology	Clinical Manifestations	Treatment
MCD	Cause of nephrotic syndrome in 90% of children and 10% of adults. Most prevalent in Asian and Caucasian populations Primary and secondary causes	Increased glomerular permeability owing to defect in cell-mediated immunity EM: Podocyte widening, effacement and shortening.	History of medication use (nonsteroidal anti-inflammatory drugs, lithium, ampicillin, sulfasalazine, bisphosphonates) hematologic malignancy, allergies/allergic reactions Onset is usually acute and can be proceeded by an infection (usually upper respiratory) approximately a week prior	Diuretics, ACEI/ARB if hypertensive and low Na diet Glucocorticoid therapy
Membranous nephropathy	Adults, most common in Caucasians. M > F with primary disease Primary and secondary causes	Autoantibodies to PLA2R targeting GBM in primary disease. Otherwise immune-complex target GBM. LM: spikes and holes EM: subepithelial deposits	Insidious onset of proteinuria and edema. Exposure to nonsteroidal anti-inflammatory drugs, penicillamine, captopril, gold, or diagnosis of hepatitis, syphilis, SLE, solid tumors, malaria.	Treat secondary cause. Otherwise, patients are monitored and risk stratified, with highest risk receiving immunosuppression (cyclophosphamide, calcineurin inhibitors, rituximab ± steroids)

(continued on next page)

Table 3
(continued)

	Demographics	Pathology	Clinical Manifestations	Treatment
FSGS	Adults. M > F and more common in Black patients Primary and secondary causes	Increased podocyte permeability, direct injury to podocytes, GBM abnormalities. Variants (ie "collapsing "in human immunodeficiency virus) exist LM: sclerosis EM: Podocyte effacement	Primary presents as nephrotic syndrome Secondary is more progressive with decreased GFR. History of heroin use, human immunodeficiency virus, Parvo B-19, hepatitis c, vesicular reflux, obesity, medications (interferon, bisphosphonates)	Primary: Immunosuppression (ie, glucocorticoids and calcineurin inhibitors) Secondary: ACEI/ARB
Diabetic nephropathy	Most common in adults More severe disease in Native Americans, Latino and Black patients	Complex interplay of inflammatory, fibrotic, hemodynamic and metabolic pathways leading to mesangial expansion, glomerular hypertrophy and sclerosis/fibrosis LM: Nodular sclerosis (Kimmelstiel Wilson)	Disease is asymptomatic early on with variable amounts of albuminuria. Decline in GFR is slow in nature. A rapid decline in GFR or rise in albumin suggests alternative cause HgbA1c may be lowered with decreased GFR. Microscopic hematuria maybe present. Urinary WBCs, red blood cell casts or dysmorphic cells suggest alternative cause.	Smoking cessation, weight loss, glycemic control, blood pressure control, ACEI or ARB SGLT2i

Amyloidosis	Genetic and secondary causes	Treatment of cause
	Fibril deposition in extracellular tissue and vascular walls. Congo red stain, apple green birefringence	*AL:* Plasma cell dyscrasia, Waldenström macroglobulinemia or non-Hodgkin lymphoma. Large amounts of proteinuria and edema, organomegaly, macroglossia, heart failure, carpal tunnel syndrome *AA:* Chronic inflammatory disease (ie, RA, IBD, chronic infections such as TB and osteomyelitis). Most commonly causes nephropathy and congestive heart failure. *Dialysis associated:* Shoulder pain and carpal tunnel syndrome *Others:* Inherited, age related, and organ specific

Abbreviations: ACEI, angiotensin-converting enzyme inhibitor; ARB, angiotensin receptor blocker; EM, electron microscopy; F, female; GBM, glomerular basement membrane; HgbA1c, hemoglobin A1c; IBD, inflammatory bowel disease; LM, light microscopy; M, male; RA, rheumatoid arthritis; SLE, systemic lupus erythematosus.

is of paramount importance. IN addition, there are other goals of therapy that can offer relief to patients from complications.

Diet

All patients with nephrotic syndrome and CKD should be on a low sodium diet. Currently, it is recommended that patients should consume less than 2400 mg of sodium per day, with hypertension recommendations at less than 1500 mg/d. This recommendation is vastly different from the usual American diet that contains more than 4000 mg of sodium per day. Patients can achieve this goal with increasing their intake of fruits and vegetables and following a diet recommended by the Dietary Approaches to Stop Hypertension Diet.[22] Processed and fast foods should be avoided owing to their high salt content.

Protein restriction has been discussed in the past for proteinuric patients, and currently that strategy is debated on true benefits of slowing CKD progression. The Kidney Disease: Improving Global Outcomes (KDIGO) guidelines suggest that protein restriction to less than 0.8 g/kg/d does not offer any advantage to lower CKD progression based on the largest trial to date (the Modification of Diet in Renal Disease study).[23] Diets that patients may already be adhering to, such as the Heart Healthy Diet or Diabetic Diet because of existing comorbidities, follow many of the same guidelines.

Hypertension

Elevated blood pressure is a cardinal sign seen in many patients with nephrotic syndrome. The retention of salt and water, activation of the renin–angiotensin–aldosterone system, and progression of kidney damage elevates blood pressure above current guidelines of goal blood pressure less than 130/80 mm Hg. The 2012 KDIGO guidelines recommend the following for proteinuric patients:

3.1.5: In both diabetic and nondiabetic adults with CKD and with urine albumin excretion of greater than 300 mg/24 hours (or equivalent*) whose office blood pressure is consistently greater than 130 mm Hg systolic or greater than 80 mm Hg diastolic treatment is aimed with blood pressure-lowering drugs to maintain a blood pressure that is consistently less than 130 mm Hg systolic and less than 80 mm Hg diastolic. (2D)

3.1.7: An angiotensin receptor blocker or angiotensin-converting enzyme inhibitor be used in both diabetic and nondiabetic adults with CKD and urine albumin excretion of greater than 300 mg/24 hours (or equivalent*). (1B)[24]

Adding a mineralocorticoid receptor antagonist with an angiotensin-converting enzyme inhibitor or angiotensin receptor blocker has shown to offer further improvement with lower blood pressure and proteinuria in the PATHWAY-2 trial.[25] In addition to the blood pressure–lowering benefit, there is evidence that renin–angiotensin–aldosterone system inhibitors limit the progression of decreased kidney function as well.[26] Patients with nephrotic syndrome are frequently overloaded with fluid and will need diuretics. Loop diuretics are the most effective inducers of diuresis in patients with reduced eGFR. These drugs are secreted into the lumen of the tubule and frequently can become bound to the albuminuria, limiting their full effectiveness compared with non-nephrotic patients. Higher doses of the diuretic are usually needed to achieve the same diuresis as patients without nephrotic syndrome. Patients with normal kidney function should start with the lowest dose of diuretic, because interpersonal response is highly variable. With decreased kidney function (estimated glomerular filtration rate of less than 60 or worse), generally it is recommended to start with double the dose of that used in a patient with a normal estimated glomerular filtration rate. There should be a low threshold to increase quickly again if diuresis is not adequate.

Edema

The physical finding of swelling in dependent areas of the body is a classic symptom in nephrotic syndrome. Aggressive diuretics are usually needed to promote the loss of salt and water. With edematous states, oral absorption of diuretics is unreliable. Intravenous infusion of loop diuretics is recommended and should be uptitrated until a desired response is seen. If a patient has chronic exposure to loop diuretics or high intravenous doses are not achieving diuresis, addition of a thiazide diuretic should be added. This process is described as sequential nephron blockade, which inactivates receptors and channels at severe points in the nephron to promote maximal diuresis. One should monitor for issues that result from urinary losses, including hypokalemia, hypomagnesemia, hypochloremic metabolic alkalosis, and azotemia with an elevated blood urea nitrogen. Ultrafiltration is a last-line option through a central venous catheter for patients who have refractory life-threatening volume overload.

A hallmark of increased proteinuria is the severity of dependent edema and anasarca. Higher proteinuria levels are associated with worse edema, although this may not be causation. Limiting proteinuria with first-line renin–angiotensin–aldosterone system inhibitor agents such as angiotensin-converting enzyme inhibitors, angiotensin receptor blockers, or mineralocorticoid receptor antagonists are recommended. Overall treatment of the root cause of the proteinuria can lead to curative elimination of the edema.

Hyperlipidemia

Elevation of lipids levels can be found in patients with all levels of proteinuria. Outside of patients with genetic hyperlipidemic conditions, patients with nephrotic syndrome can have some of the highest lipid levels. Currently, it is recommended to start patients on statin class medications to decrease cardiovascular risks, lower lipid levels, and monitor lipid levels.[27] There has been additional evidence that statins may have an impact in lowering proteinuria,[24,28] although currently there are no guidelines for ideal statins dosage to help with proteinuria. It is recommended that statin dosing follow the guidelines for dosing based on lipid response and to minimize side effects of high dosages.

COMPLICATIONS OF NEPHROTIC SYNDROME

As mentioned elsewhere in this article, one of the most worrisome complications of nephrotic syndrome is a hypercoagulopathic state, leading to both arterial and venous thrombosis. The reported incidence of deep vein thrombosis in patients with nephrotic syndrome is 15%; pulmonary embolus, 10% to 30%; and RVT in up to 37%.[29] It is hypothesized to be a result of the imbalance of glomerular loss of anticoagulants (antithrombin III) combined with increased liver procoagulant synthesis, increased platelet activation, decreased fibrinolytic activity, and localized clotting activation in the kidney vasculature. Higher risk glomerulonephritides that have been associated with thrombosis include membranous glomerulonephritis, MCD, and FSGS. Likely mechanisms are a result of these diseases being associated with the highest levels of proteinuria and high ratios of proteinuria to serum albumin. The majority of thrombotic events occur within the first 6 months of diagnosis.[30]

Hypoalbuminuria is generally accepted as having the strongest association with thromboembolism risk.[30,31] One study showed each 1.0 g/dL decrease in serum albumin resulted in an increase of venous thromboembolism of 2.13.[32] The 2012 KDIGO Clinical Practice Guideline for GN suggests that:

Anticoagulation should be considered in membranous nephropathy if any of these are present[33]:

- Serum albumin is 2.0 to 2.5 g/dL with additional risks for thrombosis (proteinuria of 10 g/d; body mass index $\geq$35 kg/m^2)
- Family history of thromboembolism with documented genetic predisposition
- New York Heart Association functional class III or IV congestive heart failure
- Recent abdominal or orthopedic surgery
- Prolonged immobilization

Current drug regimens include aspirin, low molecular weight heparin, warfarin, and direct-acting oral anticoagulants. Currently, direct-acting oral anticoagulants are not labeled for this preventative strategy by the US Food and Drug Administration. Patients with a high risk of bleeding should not be prescribed anticoagulation, but educated on their risks and symptoms to monitor for development.

Acute kidney injury is a possible side effect of nephrotic syndrome, specifically worsened in those with profound proteinuria and hypoalbuminemia.[34] The exact mechanism is poorly understood, but is believed to be from a multifactorial state of hypovolemia, interstitial edema, ischemic tubular injury, and protein droplet infiltration of the tubules and interstitium.

Other miscellaneous problems can arise from the nephrotic state. Infection risk is increased and is associated with respiratory tract infections, peritonitis, urinary tract infections, and infections related to encapsulated bacteria, including *Streptococcus pneumonia*. One contributing factor to this increased infection prevalence is hypogammaglobulinemia from proteinuria. Vitamin D loss can lead to depressed cellular immunity and increases the risk in these patients.[35] Proximal tubular dysfunction can occur with protein deposition resulting in findings such as glucosuria, phosphaturia, bicarbonaturia, and a Fanconi disease looking picture.[36] Anemia can also result from impaired synthesis of erythropoietin and should be monitored.

NEPHROLOGY CONSULTATION AND REFERRAL

Diagnosis of nephrotic syndrome is vital in helping a patient to receive appropriate treatment. The initial workup should document all physical findings and laboratory changes, including the quantification of proteinuria and albuminuria. Generally it is not recommended to begin empiric therapy of immunosuppression, because this therapy may blunt pathologic changes and can expose the patient to unnecessary toxicity. Treatment of symptoms including volume overload, hypertension, edema, and hyperlipidemia should be initiated before or during referral periods once recognized by the primary care physician.

The KDIGO workup group released guidelines recommending referral to nephrology for patients with CKD, including those with albuminuria alone.[37] If a patient has nephrotic syndrome or symptoms, an urgent nephrology consultation should be completed. Most cases of nephrotic range proteinuria, with the controversial exception of patients with diabetes, will require a kidney biopsy. Currently there does not exist a reliable noninvasive method to diagnose kidney pathology outside of a biopsy. The nephrologist may perform the kidney biopsy him or herself, or have a streamlined process to get a safe biopsy completed. Once the pathologic results are determined, the nephrologist can determine with patient's input on the best care plan.

Immunosuppression is frequently needed if enough kidney parenchyma has not succumbed to fibrosis and tubular atrophy. Anticoagulation should usually not be started in patients at high risk for thrombosis until after a biopsy is completed, unless prolonged biopsy timing is expected. A nephrologist who is up to date on current treatment guidelines will initiate an appropriate plan and may have access to clinical trials allowing patients to participate in advanced therapies. Once the treatment plan is ongoing, the patient will follow up with nephrology and continue their care with a primary care physician. Usually, the nephrologist will want to care for the patients as a team with primary care, nutrition, social work, and other health care providers.

SUMMARY

Nephrotic syndrome is an entity associated with multiple underlying etiologies and can result in ESRD; therefore, it is critical that if it is suspected, prompt referral to nephrology is initiated. Fortunately, glomerulonephritis treatments continue to evolve with delaying ESKD and transplant.

CLINICS CARE POINTS

- Nephrotic syndrome should be considered on the differential diagnosis of a patient presenting with signs and symptoms of volume overload.
- Nephrotic syndrome can be present in a patient with intact renal function, so a GFR in the normal range does not preclude the diagnosis.
- Once established as a diagnosis, complications of the nephrotic syndrome should be investigated and treated including volume overload, hypertension, and lipid abnormalities.

DISCLOSURE

The authors have nothing to disclose.

REFERENCES

1. O'Shaughnessy MM, Hogan SL, Thompson BD, et al. Glomerular disease frequencies by race, sex and region: results from the International Kidney Biopsy Survey. Nephrol Dial Transplant 2018;33(4):661–9.
2. Koye DN, Magliano DJ, Nelson RG, et al. The Global Epidemiology of Diabetes and Kidney Disease. Adv Chronic Kidney Dis 2018;25(2):121–32.
3. Rosenberg AZ, Kopp JB. Focal Segmental Glomerulosclerosis. Clin J Am Soc Nephrol 2017;12(3):502–17.
4. Sim JJ, Batech M, Hever A, et al. Distribution of Biopsy-Proven Presumed Primary Glomerulonephropathies in 2000-2011 Among a Racially and Ethnically Diverse US Population. Am J Kidney Dis 2016;68(4):533–44.
5. Couser WG. Primary Membranous Nephropathy. Clin J Am Soc Nephrol 2017;12(6):983–97.
6. Liang Y, Wan J, Chen Y, et al. Serum anti-phospholipase A2 receptor (PLA2R) antibody detected at diagnosis as a predictor for clinical remission in patients with primary membranous nephropathy: a meta-analysis. BMC Nephrol 2019;20(1). https://doi.org/10.1186/s12882-019-1544-2.
7. O'Shaughnessy MM, Hogan SL, Poulton CJ, et al. Temporal and Demographic Trends in Glomerular Disease Epidemiology in the Southeastern United States, 1986–2015. Clin J Am Soc Nephrol 2017;12(4):614–23.

8. Vivarelli M, Massella L, Ruggiero B, et al. Minimal Change Disease. Clin J Am Soc Nephrol 2017;12(2):332–45.

9. Tesar V, Zima T. Recent progress in the pathogenesis of nephrotic proteinuria. Crit Rev Clin Lab Sci 2008;45(2):139–220.

10. Svenningsen P, Friis UG, Versland JB, et al. Mechanisms of renal NaCl retention in proteinuric disease. Acta Physiol 2013;207(3):536–45.

11. van de Logt A-E, Fresquet M, Wetzels JF, et al. The anti-PLA2R antibody in membranous nephropathy: what we know and what remains a decade after its discovery. Kidney Int 2019;96(6):1292–302.

12. Johnson R, Feehally J, Floege Jurgen, et al. Comprehensive Clinical Nephrology. 6th ed. Elsevier; 2018. https://doi.org/10.1016/c2009-0-46539-5.

13. Kerlin BA, Ayoob R, Smoyer WE. Epidemiology and pathophysiology of nephrotic syndrome-associated thromboembolic disease. Clin J Am Soc Nephrol 2012; 7(3):513–20.

14. Colle JP, Mishal Z, Lesty C, et al. Abnormal fibrin clot architecture in nephrotic patients is related to hypofibrinolysis: influence of plasma biochemical modifications: a possible mechanism for the high thrombotic tendency? Thromb Haemost 1999;82(5):1482–9.

15. Mirrakhimov AE, Ali AM, Barbaryan A, et al. Primary nephrotic syndrome in adults as a risk factor for pulmonary embolism: an up-to-date review of the literature. Int J Nephrol 2014;2014:916760.

16. Agrawal S, Zaritsky JJ, Fornoni A, et al. Dyslipidaemia in nephrotic syndrome: mechanisms and treatment. Nat Rev Nephrol 2017;14(1):70.

17. Zhang LJ, Zhang Z, Li SJ, et al. Pulmonary embolism and renal vein thrombosis in patients with nephrotic syndrome: prospective evaluation of prevalence and risk factors with CT. Radiology 2014;273(3):897–906.

18. Vaziri ND. Disorders of lipid metabolism in nephrotic syndrome: mechanisms and consequences. Kidney Int 2016;90(1):41–52.

19. Ejaz S. Transcription and translation of APOL1 variants. Biosci Rep 2017;37(5). https://doi.org/10.1042/bsr20170647.

20. Baker KR, Rice L. The amyloidoses: clinical features, diagnosis and treatment. Methodist Debakey Cardiovasc J 2012;8(3):3–7.

21. Almaani S, Meara A, Rovin BH. Update on Lupus Nephritis. Clin J Am Soc Nephrol 2017;12(5):825–35.

22. CDC - Salt Home - DHDSP. 2019. Available at: https://www.cdc.gov/salt. Accessed December 25, 2019.

23. Menon V, Kopple JD, Wang X, et al. Effect of a very low-protein diet on outcomes: long-term follow-up of the Modification of Diet in Renal Disease (MDRD) Study. Am J Kidney Dis 2009;53(2):208–17.

24. Levin A, Stevens PE. Summary of KDIGO 2012 CKD Guideline: behind the scenes, need for guidance, and a framework for moving forward. Kidney Int 2014;85(1):49–61.

25. Williams B, MacDonald TM, Morant S, et al. Spironolactone versus placebo, bisoprolol, and doxazosin to determine the optimal treatment for drug-resistant hypertension (PATHWAY-2): a randomised, double-blind, crossover trial. Lancet 2015; 386(10008):2059–68.

26. Brenner BM, Cooper ME, de Zeeuw D, et al. Effects of losartan on renal and cardiovascular outcomes in patients with type 2 diabetes and nephropathy. N Engl J Med 2001;345(12):861–9.

27. Valdivielso P, Moliz M, Valera A, et al. Atorvastatin in dyslipidaemia of the nephrotic syndrome. Nephrology (Carlton) 2003;8(2):61–4.

28. Dworacka M, Krzyżagórska E, Wesołowska A, et al. Statins in low doses reduce VEGF and bFGF serum levels in patients with type 2 diabetes mellitus. Pharmacology 2014;93(1–2):32–8.
29. Glassock RJ. Prophylactic anticoagulation in nephrotic syndrome: a clinical conundrum. J Am Soc Nephrol 2007;18(8):2221–5.
30. Barbour SJ, Greenwald A, Djurdjev O, et al. Disease-specific risk of venous thromboembolic events is increased in idiopathic glomerulonephritis. Kidney Int 2012;81(2):190–5.
31. Gordon-Cappitelli J, Choi MJ. Prophylactic Anticoagulation in Adult Patients with Nephrotic Syndrome. Clin J Am Soc Nephrol 2019. https://doi.org/10.2215/cjn.05250419.
32. Lionaki S, Derebail VK, Hogan SL, et al. Venous thromboembolism in patients with membranous nephropathy. Clin J Am Soc Nephrol 2012;7(1):43–51.
33. Radhakrishnan J, Cattran DC. The KDIGO practice guideline on glomerulonephritis: reading between the (guide)lines–application to the individual patient. Kidney Int 2012;82(8):840–56.
34. Chen T, Lv Y, Lin F, et al. Acute kidney injury in adult idiopathic nephrotic syndrome. Ren Fail 2011;33(2):144–9.
35. Crew RJ, Radhakrishnan J, Appel G. Complications of the nephrotic syndrome and their treatment. Clin Nephrol 2004;62(4):245–59.
36. Vaziri ND, Kaupke CJ, Barton CH, et al. Plasma concentration and urinary excretion of erythropoietin in adult nephrotic syndrome. Pediatr Nephrol 1993;7(2):201.
37. Kidney Disease: Improving Global Outcomes (KDIGO) CKD-MBD Update Work Group. KDIGO 2017 Clinical Practice Guideline Update for the Diagnosis, Evaluation, Prevention, and Treatment of Chronic Kidney Disease–Mineral and Bone Disorder (CKD-MBD). Kidney Int Suppl 2017;7:1–59 [Errartum appears in Kidney Int Suppl 2017;7(3):e1].

Nephritic Syndrome

Perola Lamba, MD[a], Ki Heon Nam, MD[b], Jigar Contractor, MD[a],
Aram Kim, MD[a],*

KEYWORDS

- Nephritic syndrome • Infection-related glomerulonephritis • PSGN
- IgA nephropathy • Lupus nephritis • ANCA vasculitis
- Membranoproliferative glomerulonephritis • MPGN

KEY POINTS

- Nephritic syndrome is a constellation of hematuria, proteinuria, hypertension, and in some cases acute kidney injury and fluid retention characteristic of acute glomerulonephritis.
- Glomerulonephritis is characterized by glomerular injury and cellular proliferation, and can be divided into immune-mediated and pauci-immune by the presence or absence of antibody deposits.
- Treatment in acute glomerulonephritis generally targets the inflammation mediating the glomerular injury and the symptomatic clinical manifestations.
- Sporadic cases of acute glomerulonephritis progress to chronic glomerulonephritis in about 30% of adults.
- Referral to nephrology should be considered in most patients presenting with acute glomerulonephritis because it requires urgent investigation and treatment to prevent irreversible loss of kidney function.

INTRODUCTION

The glomerulus is a small, ball-shaped collection of capillaries responsible for filtering blood to make urine. Glomerulonephritis (GN) refers to a rare group of diseases that result from glomerular inflammation. Nephritic syndrome is a constellation of hematuria, proteinuria, hypertension, and in some cases acute kidney injury (AKI) and fluid retention characteristic of acute GN. GN impacts people of all ages and is responsible for 20% of chronic kidney disease cases.[1] It can be divided into immune-mediated and pauci-immune by the presence or absence of immune deposits on immunofluorescence or electron microscopy. It is essential for the primary care physician to suspect and recognize nephritic syndrome early to preserve renal function with timely

[a] Department of Medicine, Division of General Internal Medicine, Section of Hospital Medicine, Weill Cornell Medical College, 525 East 68th Street, Box 331, New York, NY 10065, USA;
[b] Department of Internal Medicine, Yonsei University Colloege of Medicine, 50 Yonsei-ro, Seodaemun-gu, Seoul, 03722, Korea
* Corresponding author.
E-mail address: ark9039@med.cornell.edu
Twitter: @jigsymd (J.C.)

Prim Care Clin Office Pract 47 (2020) 615–629
https://doi.org/10.1016/j.pop.2020.08.003
0095-4543/20/© 2020 Elsevier Inc. All rights reserved.

primarycare.theclinics.com

treatment. In this article, we review the pathophysiology, clinical manifestations, and treatment of GN as a whole and review some of the most commonly encountered GNs in primary care practice that may present with nephritic syndrome. **Table 1** highlights the key characteristics of the diseases covered in this chapter. **Box 1** summarizes the most high yield initial lab tests for the work up on nephritic syndrome.

PATHOGENESIS AND PATHOPHYSIOLOGY

GN is characterized by glomerular injury and cellular proliferation, often a result of immune-mediated inflammation. Immune-mediated injury in GN can be a result of (1) antibodies binding to intrinsic or implanted antigens within the glomerulus, or (2) deposition of circulating antigen–antibody complexes.[2] Immune complexes may be deposited in the mesangium, the subendothelial space between the endothelium and glomerular basement membrane (GBM) or the subepithelial space between the GBM and podocytes. Localization of the immune complexes depends on the charge and size of the complexes. Highly anionic molecules are excluded from the GBM and are trapped subendothelially, whereas neutral-charged molecules can accumulate in the mesangium. Subendothelial deposits tend to have more inflammatory sequelae because of the close contact with glomerular capillaries leading to increased access by leukocytes.[2]

The immune complexes activate complement and induce leukocyte infiltration of the glomerulus that produce oxygen free radicals and proteases causing GBM degradation and cellular injury. Inflammation persists until the immune-complexes are degraded by infiltrating leukocytes, mesangial cells and endogenous proteases. Resolution occurs quickly when the inciting antigen is short lived as in post-streptococcal GN (PSGN), but in chronic conditions such as lupus or viral hepatitis, inflammation may persist for prolonged periods, leading to repeated cycles of injury and proliferative GN.[2] Immune response also leads to vascular injury, platelet aggregation and activation of clotting factors leading to fibrin deposition. As a result of insults, the glomeruli respond to injury in prototypical ways, including hypercellularity, crescent formation, basement membrane thickening, hyalinosis, and sclerosis.[2]

CLINICAL MANIFESTATIONS

The typical presentation of acute GN is sudden onset of hematuria, non-nephrotic range proteinuria (<3.5 g/d), edema, hypertension and azotemia. Inflammatory insult to the glomerulus produces thinning of the GBM and formation of small pores in podocytes allowing red blood cells and protein to pass into the urine. Glomerular hematuria can be grossly evident or microscopic and is characterized by dysmorphic red blood cells and casts on urine microscopy. The inflammatory injury to the glomerulus results in decreased glomerular filtration leading to azotemia and salt and water retention producing edema, hypertension and volume overload.

TREATMENT

Therapy in acute GNs generally targets (1) the inflammation mediating the glomerular injury, and (2) the symptomatic clinical manifestations. GN may be secondary to a systemic disease, such as infection or autoimmune disease, for which managing the underlying disease is required. Immunosuppressive therapy, particularly corticosteroids, may be indicated in patients with GNs who are at high risk of progression or have rapidly worsening renal function. Supportive therapy targets improving the clinical manifestations of acute GN. Salt and water restriction along with diuretics are

Table 1
Overview of glomerulonephritides

	Demographics	Pathology	Clinical Manifestations	Treatment
IRGN	Children ill developing countries Elderly in developed countries	Immune complex deposition on epithelial side of GBM appearing as dense deposits	Most cases subclinical. Low C3, CH50. *PSGN:* follows infection by weeks. Increase in antistreptolysin O titer. *Nonstreptococcal bacterial infectious GN:* infection is concurrent.	*PSGN:* Prophylaxis for cohabitants *Nonstreptococcal bacterial infectious GN:* Treat underlying infection
IgAN	Higher incidence in people of Caucasian ancestry Male > female	Excess IgA production with deposits of circulating IgA complexes or IgA binding of in situ antigens *IgAV:* leukocytoclastic vasculitis of capillary walls	Recurrent gross hematuria concurrent with upper respiratory infection 10% with acute GN. *IgAV:* lower limb palpable purpura, abdominal pain, proteinuria/hematuria, acute arthritis/arthralgias.	ACEi/ARBs; Corticosteroids for refractory, proteinuria; Monitor for hematuria and worsening renal function annually *RPGN:* induction with steroids or CP followed by AZA maintenance
LN	Female >> male Higher incidence in urban settings and in people of African, Hispanic, and Asian Ancestry	*I* mesangial immune deposits on electron microscopy and immunofluorescence only *II:* mesangial hypercellularity and matrix expansion *III:* GN involving <50% of glomeruli with subendothelial deposits *IV:* GN involving >50% of glomeruli with diffuse subendothelial deposits *V:* global or segmental immune deposits, may occur in combination with class *II* or *IV* *VI:* > 90% of glomeruli are globally sclerosed	Systemic SLE manifestations. *I/II:* minimal manifestations. *III/IV:* low complement, high anti-dsDNA titers; 1/3 with nephrotic range proteinuria; active urine sediment; AKI very common. *V:* nephrotic syndrome. *VI:* slowly progressive renal failure, bland urine sediment.	*I/II:* supportive care. Steroids or CNI if proteinuria >3 g/d *III/IV:* 6 mo induction with steroids + MMF or CP; maintenance with MMF or AZA *V:* Steroids + MMF *VI:* Supportive care to slow progression

(continued on next page)

Table 1
(continued)

	Demographics	Pathology	Clinical Manifestations	Treatment
MPGN	Rare May be secondary to infections, autoimmune or myeloproliferative disorders	Mesangial hypercellularity and deposits of complement ± immune complexes producing capillary wall thickening and GBM duplication Dysregulation of the alternative pathway of complement in C3 glomerulonephropathy. *Immune complex-mediated MPGN:* Ig-positive, complement-positive *C3 glomerulopathy:* Ig-negative, complement-positive	Variable timing and severity of clinical manifestations. *Primary immune complex mediated:* no causal agent. *Secondary immune complex mediated:* infections - bacteria, fungi and viruses (hepatitis B/C); autoimmune - mixed cryoglobulinemia. SLE, Sjogren's syndrome, or rheumatoid arthritis; malignancy - myeloma. B-cell lymphoma, and chronic lymphocytic leukemia.	Treat underlying cause Mild: supportive care, particularly in children; Can consider low dose steroids Severe: immunosuppressive agents like CP, CNI, rituximab. and steroids; sometimes plasmapheresis
AAV	Male = female Older white adults Rare in children	ANCA-activated neutrophils cause small vessel inflammation that disrupt vessel walls causing local fibrinous necrosis and crescent formation; GPA associated PR-3-ANCA and MPA associated MPO-ANCA	Involvement of ear, nose, throat, upper airways, lungs, kidneys, eyes, nervous system and skin with overlap between GPA/MPA; ANCA+ supports diagnosis.	Induction: steroids + CP or rituximab; Plasmapheresis for pulmonary hemorrhage or severe renal injury; Maintenance: AZA for 12 mo

Abbreviation: GN, glomerulonephritis.

Box 1
Laboratory workup for nephritic syndrome

- Urinalysis with microscopy
- Spot urine protein:creatinine ratio
- Complete blood count
- Comprehensive metabolic panel
- Erythrocyte sedimentation rate/C-reactive protein
- Complement panel
- Anti-streptolysin O
- Hepatitis B and C serologies
- Serum and urine electrophoresis immunofixation
- Serum free light chain
- ANA with titer
- ANCA (P-ANCA, c-ANCA)
- Anti-GBM

---

mainstays to improve edema and hypertension, but occasionally antihypertensive medications are required.

PROGNOSIS

The prognosis in nephritic syndrome depends on the causative disease and the age at which one develops GN. Typically children fare better and are more likely to have complete recovery compared with adults. Sporadic cases of acute GN progress to chronic GN in about 30% of adults and only 10% of children. GN is responsible for 16% of all end-stage renal disease (ESRD) cases in the United States and is one of the leading causes of ESRD in children and adolescents.[1] Although recurrence is not common, it is more likely in adults and more often leads to end-stage kidney disease necessitating dialysis or transplantation. Clinical factors such as nephrotic range proteinuria, elevated serum creatinine, and hypertension are associated with worse outcomes.

INFECTION-RELATED GLOMERULONEPHRITIS

Infection-related GN (IRGN) is triggered by an infectious antigen, most commonly streptococcus, but bacterial (eg, staphylococcal endocarditis, pneumococcal pneumonia and meningococcemia), viral (eg, hepatitis B, hepatitis C, mumps, human immunodeficiency virus, varicella and infectious mononucleosis) and parasitic (malaria, toxoplasmosis) infections are increasingly recognized.[3] IRGN typically affects children aged 2 to 14 years in underdeveloped countries, but more frequently impacts the elderly in developed countries.[4] In adults, most IRGNs occur in subacute or chronic infections with prolonged antigenemia, as there is a greater opportunity for pathogen-directed immune complexes to form in the circulation. Pathologically, immune complexes deposit in the glomeruli and activate complement. Histopathology reveals enlarged, hypercellular glomeruli, obliterated capillaries, interstitial edema, red cell casts, and crescent formation in severe cases. On immunofluorescence, granular deposits of IgG, IgM and C3 are seen in the mesangium and along the GBM. On electron microscopy, there are discrete, amorphous electron dense immune complex deposits that look like humps primarily on the epithelial side of the GBM.[2] The clinical spectrum can vary widely, from asymptomatic microscopic hematuria to fulminant nephritic syndrome with oliguric renal failure.[1]

Poststreptococcal Glomerulonephritis

PSGN is the prototypical IRGN where GN is preceded by group A beta-hemolytic streptococcal pharyngeal or skin infection. The latent period between onset of infection and nephritis is 1 to 3 weeks for pharyngitis and 2 to 6 weeks for skin infections, which is likely the time required to produce immune complexes. PSGN was common, especially among children, but with improved hand hygiene and widespread antibiotic use, the incidence has dramatically decreased in developed countries.[4] The global incidence of PSGN is estimated to be 470,000 cases per year, the majority of which are in low- and middle-income countries. Care must be taken with family members as PSGN can impact 40% of cohabitants and outbreaks of PSGN in developed countries are often due to skin infections.[5]

The majority of cases are subclinical, but the prototypical presentation of acute GN is commonly seen. Hematuria is present in nearly all cases and 30% to 50% of cases have macroscopic hematuria.[6] Moderate hypertension is commonplace, whereas hypertensive encephalopathy and oliguric AKI requiring dialysis are rare but serious complications.

Because the infection precedes the presentation of PSGN, throat and skin cultures are unreliable to diagnose recent streptococcal infection. However, an elevated antistreptolysin O titer is found in up to 90% of patients. More importantly, it is the increase in titer rather than the absolute level that is specific for the diagnosis of PSGN.[6] Serum levels of C4 are usually normal whereas C3 and CH50 are nearly always depressed during the first weeks and return to normal in 8 to 10 weeks.[3]

Antibiotic therapy for streptococcal infection is indicated for all patients and their cohabitants to prevent the spread of infection.[4] Although antibiotics are indicated, there is no evidence to suggest antibiotics prevent or alter the course of PSGN after the onset of symptoms. Typically, immunosuppressive therapy is not used and, in the absence of hypertension and oliguria, PSGN can be managed as an outpatient with symptomatic therapy.

Most patients, particularly children, with PSGN do well, but about 1% will go on to develop chronic kidney disease.[7] In the short term, most patients begin to recover in a week after the onset of symptoms with hypertension and fluid retention improving first, although proteinuria and microscopic hematuria may persist for months to years.[7] Recurrence is uncommon, but some, particularly adults with underlying renal disease, may develop recurrent GN.

Non–Streptococcal Bacterial Infection-Related Glomerulonephritis

The most common cause of nonstreptococcal bacterial infectious GN is *Staphylococcus aureus*, but notably gram-negative bacteria account for 10% of cases. In contrast with PSGN, most infection is concurrent with GN in nonstreptococcal bacterial infectious GN.[8] The clinical manifestations are similar to PSGN, but tend to be more aggressive with nephrotic range proteinuria, hypertension, heart failure, and AKI occurring more frequently. Extrarenal manifestations are uncommon, but purpuric skin rash may occur in a subset of patients with staphylococcal-associated GN.[8]

Low C3 is present in 35% to 80% of patients and normalizes within 2 months of the resolution of the infectious trigger.[9] Anti–neutrophil cytoplasmic antibody (ANCA) seropositivity may occur, especially with endocarditis.[9]

Less than one-half of patients with nonstreptococcal bacterial infectious GN have complete resolution of azotemia and proteinuria and mortality rates can exceed 10%, even in those with histopathologic resolution of GN.[10] Recovery from nonstreptococcal infectious GN depends on the causative organism, comorbidities, severity of disease, and our ability to treat the underlying infection. Older age, a history of diabetic kidney disease, and glomerular scarring, as evidenced by heavy proteinuria, severe hypertension, and persistent azotemia, predispose to worse outcomes.[10]

IgA NEPHROPATHY

IgA nephropathy (IgAN) is a systemic disease that results in mesangial IgA deposition causing immune-mediated injury. It is more common in men in their teens and twenties and is the most frequently diagnosed GN in adults, but still rare with an annual global incidence of 2.5 per 100,000 people.[11] In rare instances IgAN has been shown to have a genetic component, but no single causal gene has been identified.[4]

IgAN results from mucosal plasma cells overproducing IgA1 often with galactose deficiency in side chains near the hinge region of the heavy chain. These IgA1 molecules self-aggregate and form antigen–antibody complexes with IgA and IgG directed at the IgA1 hinge region leading to deposit formation in the mesangial space.[12] Then, complexed galactose deficient IgA complexes activate the mesangial cells leading to increased expression of proinflammatory and profibrotic cytokines and growth factors. The Oxford Score rates the severity of 4 reliably identifiable histopathologic findings to create a universal score that predicts poor kidney outcomes independent of, and in addition to, clinical outcomes. The Oxford score assesses the presence and severity of mesangial hypercellularity, segmental glomerulosclerosis, endocapillary hypercellularity, and tubular atrophy or interstitial fibrosis on biopsy.[13,14]

The clinical presentation of IgAN is also variable, ranging from asymptomatic microscopic hematuria to rapidly progressive GN (RPGN). Less than 10% of patients with IgAN will present with nephritic syndrome. IgAN typically presents as recurrent episodes of gross hematuria during an upper respiratory infection or asymptomatic microscopic hematuria on routine screening. Approximately one-half of IgAN patients younger than age 40 will have macroscopic hematuria at the time of their initial presentation.[8,15] The presence of nephrotic range proteinuria suggests widespread proliferative GN or an overlap syndrome with minimal change nephropathy.

Serum IgA levels are elevated in up to 50% of patients with IgAN, but lacks sufficient specificity. Because there are no specific diagnostic laboratory studies, kidney biopsy with immunofluorescence or immunoperoxidase studies for IgA deposits is necessary for the diagnosis of IgAN. Symptomatic treatment and prevention of worsening renal function is the foundation of treatment in IgAN and typically is sufficient in those with mild or moderate disease. Angiotensin-converting enzyme inhibitors (ACEi) and angiotensin receptor blockers (ARB) are used to manage hypertension and proteinuria. An unacceptably high risk of hyperkalemia precludes using both ACEi and ARBs concurrently. The role of corticosteroids is not well-described, and treatment is not without risk, such as immunosuppression and Cushing syndrome.[11] Thus, corticosteroids are generally reserved for patients with progressively worsening renal function or persistent proteinuria of more than 1 g/d despite maximal ACEi or ARB therapy. For rapidly progressive IgAN, immunosuppressive therapy is warranted and consists of induction with corticosteroids and cyclophosphamide (CP) followed by maintenance therapy with azathioprine (AZA).[5] Currently, there is not enough data to recommend mycophenolate or rituximab.[11] The impact of fish oil containing omega-3 fatty acids on renal outcomes has conflicting data. Patients with IgAN should be monitored annually for worsening renal function, hematuria, and proteinuria; over the course of 20 years, 30% of patients with IgAN will develop progressive proteinuria and glomerular insufficiency.[16] The likelihood of adverse renal outcomes in IgAN depends on the degree of proteinuria, hypertension, histopathologic findings, and the glomerular filtration rate at diagnosis and during follow-up. The severity of proteinuria is the single most important predictor of renal outcomes in IgAN. Those with a limited duration and degree of proteinuria have a low risk of progressive kidney disease, whereas those with proteinuria of greater than 1 g/d have increased risk with the highest risk in those with proteinuria of greater than 3 to 4 g/d.[17,18]

LUPUS NEPHRITIS

Systemic lupus erythematosus (SLE) is caused by an aberrant autoimmune response to nuclear autoantigens. Genetic, hormonal, and environmental factors influence the loss of self-tolerance, leading to nonspecific activation of autoreactive B cells and production of polyclonal antibodies, allowing immune complexes containing anti-DNA antibodies to form.[19] Immune complex deposits in the GBM, subendothelial, mesangial, and subepithelial areas lead to an augmented innate immune response characterized by complement activation and leukocyte infiltration. The resulting damage to the renal parenchyma triggers healing responses that further exacerbate renal injury. The overall incidence of SLE ranges from 1.8 to 7.6 cases per 100,000 annually, and the prevalence ranges from 4 to 250 per 100,000 people, with up to a 12-fold female preponderance.[20] At the time of diagnosis, nearly one-half will have lupus nephritis (LN), and 60% will develop clinically relevant GN during the course of their illness.[4] The prevalence of LN is higher in urban settings and in people of African, Hispanic, and Asian ancestry.[21] Further, black and Hispanic patients have worse outcomes with LN.

The clinical manifestations of LN are often subtle and frequently discovered by screening urinalysis and serum creatinine measurement. The most common finding in LN is proteinuria, but hematuria, active urine sediment with red blood cell casts, hypertension, and renal failure may also be present. Therefore, all patients with a known or suspected diagnosis of SLE should undergo urinalysis screening at regular intervals even in the absence of symptoms and, if abnormal, histopathology should be used to confirm the diagnosis.[22]

Clinical presentations, treatment, and prognosis of LN are closely linked to renal pathology. The Renal Pathology Society/International Society of Nephrology classification was developed in 2004, dividing LN into 6 classes based on clinicopathologic correlations. Occasionally with relapses and flares, there may be progression of LN, and if rebiopsied these patients may demonstrate proliferative or fibrotic disease, thereby altering prognosis and treatment.[22]

Class I (Minimal Mesangial) and II (Mesangial Proliferative) Lupus Nephritis

Patients with class I and II LN often have minimal evidence of renal disease with minimal proteinuria, microscopic hematuria, inactive urine sediment, and a normal serum creatinine.[23] As a result, class I and II LN are rarely diagnosed. No immunosuppressive treatment is required, because the vast majority of these patients will have a benign long-term course.[24,25] However, for patients with class II LN with significant proteinuria (>3 g/d), glucocorticoids or calcineurin inhibitors (CNI) are recommended.

Class III (Focal) and IV (Diffuse) Lupus Nephritis

Patients with class III and IV LN typically have low complement levels and high anti-DNA antibody titers. Patients with class III LN have hypertension, hematuria with active urine sediment, proteinuria that may be in the nephrotic range in up to one-third of patients, and elevated serum creatinine in nearly one-quarter of patients. Class IV LN is the most common histologic pattern and the most severe form of LN. Virtually all patients with class IV LN have hematuria and proteinuria. Renal dysfunction, hypertension, and nephrotic syndrome are also common.[26] Early biopsy is important, because delays in diagnosis and treatment significantly increase the risk of renal failure.[27] Even with treatment, one-quarter of patients will have progressive worsening of renal function at 3 years and by 10 years nearly 20% require dialysis or transplantation.[27] During the course of the disease, the number and severity of renal relapses, particularly those associated with an increase in serum creatinine, are risk factors for progression, whereas improvement of clinical manifestations such as proteinuria are associated with improved kidney outcomes.[28,29]

Class III and IV LN require immunosuppressive treatment. Induction therapy is typically 6 months of corticosteroids and either CP or mycophenolate mofetil (MMF), which have similar efficacy in achieving remission. If there is no response by 6 months or clinical worsening, most guidelines recommend changing the immunosuppressive agent. AZA and CNI are second-line induction agents. Maintenance therapy is indicated in all patients after induction with either MMF and AZA. Most studies find no significant difference in efficacy between MMF and AZA, although MMF may be associated with a lower rate of treatment failure, renal flares, and side effects.[30] Increasingly, CNI may be considered as an alternative therapy given their promising efficacy and adverse effect profile.[31]

Class V (Membranous) Lupus Nephritis

Patients with class V LN typically present with nephrotic syndrome with proteinuria and edema. Some patients may also have microscopic hematuria, hypertension, venous thromboembolism and renal dysfunction.[32] Class V LN is associated with a good prognosis and is typically managed without immunosuppressive therapy. Patients with worsening renal function or proteinuria in the nephrotic range should be treated with corticosteroids plus an additional immunosuppressive agent including CP, CNI, MMF, or AZA. The mainstay of therapy is management of hypertension, edema, and proteinuria with ACEIs or ARBs used as first-line agents.

Class VI (Advanced Sclerosing) Lupus Nephritis

Class VI LN is the result of burned out LN of long duration.[23] Patients with class VI LN usually have slowly progressive renal dysfunction with proteinuria and bland urine sediment. Class VI should not be treated aggressively because the renal prognosis is poor despite treatment. Management should focus on therapies to slow the progression of renal disease.[21]

MEMBRANOPROLIFERATIVE GLOMERULONEPHRITIS

Membranoproliferative GN (MPGN) is a rare group of glomerular diseases characterized by mesangial hypercellularity and subendothelial deposition of complement and sometimes immune complexes, resulting in thickening of glomerular capillary walls and basement membrane duplication.[33] Immunofluorescence staining is used to classify MPGN into 2 types, immune complex–mediated MPGN and complement-mediated MPGN (C3 glomerulopathy [C3G]). All types stain positive for C3 complement and hypocomplementemia is common. Notably, however, C3G does not stain for immunoglobulins.[34] MPGN is more common in children and in underdeveloped nations.

In immune complex-mediated MPGN, circulating immune complexes with a triggering antigen are deposited in glomerular capillaries and mesangium, activating complement and attracting inflammatory cells. The proliferative response creates a new basement membrane, trapping the immune complexes and causing a double contouring of the GBM on light microscopy. Hyperlobulation of the glomerular tufts results from an infiltration of mononuclear cells and an increase in mesangial cells and mesangial matrix.[33] In C3G, dysregulation of the alternative pathway of complement occurs through hereditary or acquired defects. It is commonly associated with a circulating autoantibody called C3 nephritic factor, which binds to and stabilizes C3 convertase.[35]

MPGN has a variable clinical presentation, ranging from asymptomatic hematuria and proteinuria to acute GN, nephrotic syndrome, chronic kidney disease, and even RPGN.[36] The degree of renal insufficiency is variable and hypertension may or may not be present. Secondary immune complex-mediated MPGN may be associated with systemic disease or infection, including viral infections such as hepatitis B or C, and autoimmune diseases such as mixed cryoglobulinemia, SLE, Sjogren's syndrome, and scleroderma. Myeloproliferative disorders such as monoclonal gammopathy of undetermined significance, chronic lymphocytic leukemia, low-grade B-cell lymphomas, and multiple myeloma may also cause MPGN owing to deposition of monoclonal immunoglobulins in the mesangium and glomerular capillary walls. Therefore, a careful evaluation for infections, autoimmune diseases, and myeloproliferative disorders is warranted. Despite improvement of diagnostic modalities, idiopathic remains the most frequent etiology of immune complex-mediated MPGN, followed by bacterial infections, viral infections, autoimmune diseases, and hematologic malignancies.[37]

The prognosis in MPGN depends on the severity of disease rather than its histopathologic class, but likely the most important prognostic factor is the ability to ascertain the precipitating cause and prescribe effective treatment. For idiopathic immune complex-mediated MPGN, treatment remains unclear. For mild disease, particularly children with non-nephrotic proteinuria, supportive treatment may be sufficient. For severe disease, immunosuppressive drugs including CP, CNI, rituximab, and steroids, as well as plasmapheresis, have been used. Low-dose glucocorticoids have been shown to improve renal survival in children, but it is unclear whether similar effects are achieved in adults.[5,38] Historically, idiopathic MPGN has had worse prognosis than secondary MPGN, but this result may be reflective of ineffective diagnostics in determining the precipitating etiology of MPGN. In idiopathic MPGN, only about 20% of patients will have resolution of their proteinuria, whereas most patients will have progressive worsening of renal function. At 10 years, more than one-half of patients will have developed ESRD, an estimated 70% will have ESRD by 20 years, and nearly 50% of patients who undergo transplant will have a recurrence of MPGN.[39]

If immune complex-mediated MPGN is secondary to a precipitating event, resolution of GN follows treatment of the underlying cause. For instance, antiviral therapy to treat viral hepatitis, antibiotics for bacterial endocarditis, or chemotherapy for malignancy can produce partial or complete remission.[40]

In C3G, a small number of cases report promising results for eculizumab, a monoclonal antibody that binds to the C5 proteins in the complement cascade. However, additional studies are necessary to assess the full spectrum of benefits and risks.[34]

ANTINEUTROPHIL CYTOPLASMIC ANTIBODY–ASSOCIATED VASCULITIS

ANCA-associated vasculitis (AAV) is a group of small vessel vasculitides characterized by the scarcity of immunoglobulin deposits in vessel walls, and includes granulomatosis with polyangiitis (GPA) and microscopic polyangiitis (MPA). Characteristically, AAV has antibodies directed to myeloperoxidase (MPO) and proteinase 3 (PR3), antigens typically found in the granules of neutrophils and lysosomes of monocytes.[41] MPO-ANCA positivity is generally associated with MPA, whereas PR3-ANCA positivity is associated with GPA.

AAV is most frequently seen in older white adults in their 50s and 60s with an even gender distribution and is rare in children and young adults. The cumulative incidence is less than 1 per 100,000 with GPA diagnosed much more frequently than MPA; the prevalence is 2.5 per 100,000 with an equal distribution between GPA and MPA. As diagnosis and treatments for GPA and MPA improve over time, so have mortality and ESRD rates.[42] Despite these improvements, 1 in 4 patients will develop ESRD.[43]

The pathogenesis of AAV is multifactorial with a complex interplay between genetic and environmental factors and characteristics of innate and adaptive immune systems. During cell death, nuclear DNA and cytoplasmic proteins like MPO and PR3 are extruded into the extracellular space activating the immune system and neutrophils. ANCA-activated neutrophils penetrate the vessel walls, activate complement, and activate the coagulation cascade to produce fibrinoid necrosis and glomerular crescents. Over time, the acute inflammation and necrosis is replaced by collagen from infiltrating macrophages, lymphocytes and activated fibroblasts producing sclerosis.[44]

AAV is a systemic small vessel vasculitis with diffuse manifestations that impact the integumentary, pulmonary, nervous and renal systems. Constitutional symptoms may precede organ involvement by weeks to months.[23] There is significant overlap in the clinical presentation of GPA and MPA, but a distinguishing feature is that MPA lacks granulomatous manifestations.[45] Ear, nose, and throat abnormalities like nasal crusting, oral ulcers, and sinusitis are common in GPA, whereas peripheral nervous system abnormalities are common in MPA. However, no single clinical feature is diagnostic of GPA or MPA.

Renal involvement is common in both GPA and MPA. GPA on average tends to present with milder disease with microscopic hematuria and non-nephrotic proteinuria, whereas RPGN is a common feature of MPA. However, renal manifestations of both diseases cannot be distinguished by severity or time course, as cases of RPGN with GPA and indolent presentations with MPA are seen. Some patients will have renal-limited GPA without involvement of other organs, further complicating the diagnosis of AAV.[45]

A positive test for ANCA strongly supports the diagnosis of AAV, although both false-positive and false-negative results may be seen. PR3-ANCA is present in more than 90% of patients with generalized forms of GPA and in 50% to 80% of patients with limited forms of the disease.[46] Twenty percent of patients with GPA have MPO-ANCA; however, MPO-ANCA is more commonly associated with MPA (60%) or renal-limited vasculitis (80%). Furthermore, 5% of patients with GPA are ANCA negative.[45] Additionally, 30% of patients with MPA have PR3-ANCA, and 10% are ANCA negative. There are no routine laboratory tests that are specific for AAV, although leukocytosis, thrombocytosis, anemia, and elevated inflammatory markers may be observed. ANA, serum complement levels, and cryoglobulins tend to be normal.[23]

Treatment is initiated to limit further inflammatory injury and consists of induction therapy with corticosteroids and an immunosuppressive agent followed by maintenance therapy with AZA for 1 year. Untreated GPA and MPA have mortality rates approaching 90% and even with treatment mortality rates are still elevated.[42,47] Prednisone is typically started at 1 mg/kg/d with maximum daily dose of 60 mg, and then tapered over 3 to 4 months. CP is the typical immunosuppressive agent used in AAV, but rituximab is a noninferior alternative.[48,49] CP can be given as a daily oral regimen or as an intravenous monthly pulse. The monthly pulse regimen provides a lower total cumulative dose and is the preferred choice, because the risk of malignancy with CP is dose dependent. Plasmapheresis may be added as adjunctive therapy for patients with pulmonary hemorrhage or severe renal disease at presentation. Once remission is achieved with CP or rituximab, it is safe and effective to switch to AZA for the duration of maintenance therapy, which is typically 12 months, but the optimal duration is unknown. The adverse prognosis in GPA and MPA is not only due to pulmonary, cardiovascular, and renal injury, but also from prolonged immunosuppressive therapy, which increases the risk of infections and malignancy.[42,43]

NEPHROLOGY CONSULT AND REFERRAL

A nephrology consult should be considered for most patients presenting with acute GN because it requires urgent investigation and treatment to prevent irreversible loss of kidney function. It is especially important in patients with RPGN, where prompt diagnosis and treatment are essential. Therefore, the primary care physician must rapidly recognize the syndrome and make an urgent referral for biopsy and treatment. Renal biopsy is indicated for most patients with suspected GN, except perhaps in children with a clear diagnosis of PSGN, because the disease is generally self-limited and histopathology is unlikely to alter therapy. After the initiation of therapy, biopsy should be considered in cases of relapses or worsening renal function, because a change in histopathology may impact treatment and prognosis. In cases of progressive worsening of renal function to ESRD, a referral for dialysis or transplantation should be made according to local standards of care.

SUMMARY

Nephritic syndrome is an entity caused by substantial inflammatory damage to the glomerular system and is associated with multiple underlying etiologies, typically characterized by hematuria, proteinuria, hypertension, and in some cases AKI and fluid retention. The prognosis depends on the underlying cause; therefore, the initiation of a prompt workup is crucial to prevent irreversible loss of kidney function.

DISCLOSURE

The authors have nothing to disclose.

REFERENCES

1. Centers for Disease Control and Prevention. Chronic kidney disease in the United States, 2019. Atlanta (GA): US Department of Health and Human Services, Centers for Disease Control and Prevention; 2019.
2. Kumar V, Abbas A, Aster J. Robbins & Cotran pathologic basis of disease (Robbins Pathology). 9th edition. Philadelphia: Elsevier; 2015. p. 1408.
3. Chapter 9: Infection-related glomerulonephritis. Kidney Int Suppl 2011;2(2): 200–8.

4. Longo DL, Kasper DL, Jameson JL, et al, editors. Harrison's principles of internal medicine. 18th edition. McGraw Hill Medical; 2012.

5. Primary glomerular diseases. In: Clarkson M, Brenner B, Magee C, editors. Pocket guide to Brenner and Rector's the kidney. 2nd edition. Philadelphia, PA: Elsevier; 2011. p. 222–49.

6. Hunt EAK, Somers MJG. Infection-related glomerulonephritis. Pediatr Clin North Am 2019;66(1):59–72.

7. Rodriguez-Iturbe B, Musser JM. The current state of poststreptococcal glomerulonephritis. J Am Soc Nephrol 2008;19(10):1855 64.

8. Satoskar AA, Parikh SV, Nadasdy T. Epidemiology, pathogenesis, treatment and outcomes of infection-associated glomerulonephritis. Nat Rev Nephrol 2020; 16(1):32–50.

9. Nasr SH, Radhakrishnan J, D'Agati VD. Bacterial infection-related glomerulonephritis in adults. Kidney Int 2013;83(5):792–803.

10. Wang S-Y, Bu R, Zhang Q, et al. Clinical, pathological, and prognostic characteristics of glomerulonephritis related to staphylococcal infection. Medicine (Baltimore) 2016;95(15):e3386.

11. Rodrigues JC, Haas M, Reich HN. IgA Nephropathy. Clin J Am Soc Nephrol 2017; 12(4):677–86.

12. Wyatt RJ, Julian BA. IgA nephropathy. N Engl J Med 2013;368(25):2402–14.

13. Working Group of the International IgA Nephropathy Network and the Renal Pathology Society, Cattran DC, Coppo R, Cook HT, et al. The Oxford classification of IgA nephropathy: rationale, clinicopathological correlations, and classification. Kidney Int 2009;76(5):534–45.

14. Working Group of the International IgA Nephropathy Network and the Renal Pathology Society, Roberts ISD, Cook HT, Troyanov S, et al. The Oxford classification of IgA nephropathy: pathology definitions, correlations, and reproducibility. Kidney Int 2009;76(5):546–56.

15. Saha MK, Pendergraft WF, Jennette JC, et al. Primary glomerular disease. In: Skorecki K, Chertow GM, Marsden PA, et al, editors. Brenner & rector's the kidney [electronic resource]. Philadelphia: Elsevier; 2020. p. 1007–91.

16. Rekola S, Bergstrand A, Bucht H. Deterioration of GFR in IgA nephropathy as measured by 51Cr-EDTA clearance. Kidney Int 1991;40(6):1050–4.

17. Berthoux F, Mohey H, Laurent B, et al. Predicting the risk for dialysis or death in IgA nephropathy. J Am Soc Nephrol 2011;22(4):752–61.

18. Bartosik LP, Lajoie G, Sugar L, et al. Predicting progression in IgA nephropathy. Am J Kidney Dis 2001;38(4):728–35.

19. Lech M, Anders H-J. The pathogenesis of lupus nephritis. J Am Soc Nephrol 2013;24(9):1357–66.

20. Singh S, Saxena R. Lupus nephritis. Am J Med Sci 2009;337(6):451–60.

21. Anvari E, Provenzano LF, Nevares A, et al. Lupus nephritis (including antiphospholipid antibody syndrome), adult. In: Trachtman H, Hogan J, Herlitz L, et al, editors. Glomerulonephritis. Cham (Switzerland): Springer; 2019.

22. Almaani S, Meara A, Rovin BH. Update on lupus nephritis. Clin J Am Soc Nephrol 2017;12(5):825–35.

23. Radhakrishnan J, Appel GB, D'Agati VD. Secondary glomerular disease. In: Skorecki K, Chertow GM, Marsden PA, et al, editors. Brenner & rector's the kidney [electronic resource]. Philadelphia: Elsevier; 2020. p. 1092–164.

24. Hahn BH, McMahon MA, Wilkinson A, et al. American College of Rheumatology guidelines for screening, treatment, and management of lupus nephritis. Arthritis Care Res (Hoboken) 2012;64(6):797–808.

25. Bertsias GK, Tektonidou M, Amoura Z, et al. Joint European League Against Rheumatism and European Renal Association-European Dialysis and Transplant Association (EULAR/ERA-EDTA) recommendations for the management of adult and paediatric lupus nephritis. Ann Rheum Dis 2012;71(11):1771–82.
26. Bomback AS, Appel GB. Updates on the treatment of lupus nephritis. J Am Soc Nephrol 2010;21(12):2028–35.
27. Faurschou M, Starklint H, Halberg P, et al. Prognostic factors in lupus nephritis: diagnostic and therapeutic delay increases the risk of terminal renal failure. J Rheumatol 2006;33(8):1563–9.
28. Appel GB, Cohen DJ, Pirani CL, et al. Long-term follow-up of patients with lupus nephritis. A study based on the classification of the World Health Organization. Am J Med 1987;83(5):877–85.
29. Korbet SM, Lewis EJ, Schwartz MM, et al. Factors predictive of outcome in severe lupus nephritis. Lupus Nephritis Collaborative Study Group. Am J Kidney Dis 2000;35(5):904–14.
30. Dooley MA, Jayne D, Ginzler EM, et al. Mycophenolate versus azathioprine as maintenance therapy for lupus nephritis. N Engl J Med 2011;365(20):1886–95.
31. Lee YH, Song GG. Comparative efficacy and safety of tacrolimus, mycophenolate mofetil, azathioprine, and cyclophosphamide as maintenance therapy for lupus nephritis: a Bayesian network meta-analysis of randomized controlled trials. Z Rheumatol 2016;76(10):904–12.
32. Sloan RP, Schwartz MM, Korbet SM, et al. Long-term outcome in systemic lupus erythematosus membranous glomerulonephritis. Lupus Nephritis Collaborative Study Group. J Am Soc Nephrol 1996;7(2):299–305.
33. Sethi S, Nester CM, Smith RJH. Membranoproliferative glomerulonephritis and C3 glomerulopathy: resolving the confusion. Kidney Int 2012;81(5):434–41.
34. Masani N, Jhaveri KD, Fishbane S. Update on membranoproliferative GN. Clin J Am Soc Nephrol 2014;9(3):600–8.
35. Cook HT, Pickering MC. Histopathology of MPGN and C3 glomerulopathies. Nat Rev Nephrol 2015;11(1):14–22.
36. Sethi S, Fervenza FC. Membranoproliferative glomerulonephritis–a new look at an old entity. N Engl J Med 2012;366(12):1119–31.
37. Pavinic J, Miglinas M. The incidence of possible causes of membranoproliferative glomerulonephritis: a single-center experience. Hippokratia 2015;19(4):314–8.
38. Diaz MM, Sans L, Arce Y, et al. Membranoproliferative or mesangiocapillary glomerulonephritis. In: Shoenfeld Y, Cervera R, Gershwin EM, editors. Diagnostic criteria in autoimmune diseases. Humana Press; 2008. p. 503–6.
39. Little MA, Dupont P, Campbell E, et al. Severity of primary MPGN, rather than MPGN type, determines renal survival and post-transplantation recurrence risk. Kidney Int 2006;69(3):504–11.
40. Elewa U, Sandri AM, Kim WR, et al. Treatment of hepatitis B virus-associated nephropathy. Nephron Clin Pract 2011;119(1):c41–9 [discussion c49].
41. Xiao H, Hu P, Falk RJ, et al. Overview of the Pathogenesis of ANCA-Associated Vasculitis. Kidney Dis (Basel) 2016;1(4):205–15.
42. Mun CH, Yoo J, Jung SM, et al. The initial predictors of death in 153 patients with ANCA-associated vasculitis in a single Korean centre. Clin Exp Rheumatol 2018; 36 Suppl 111(2):65–72.
43. Lionaki S, Hogan SL, Jennette CE, et al. The clinical course of ANCA small-vessel vasculitis on chronic dialysis. Kidney Int 2009;76(6):644–51.
44. Jennette JC, Nachman PH. ANCA glomerulonephritis and vasculitis. Clin J Am Soc Nephrol 2017;12(10):1680–91.

45. Geetha D, Jefferson JA. ANCA-associated vasculitis: core curriculum 2020. Am J Kidney Dis 2019. https://doi.org/10.1053/j.ajkd.2019.04.031.
46. Ponte C, Águeda AF, Luqmani RA. Clinical features and structured clinical evaluation of vasculitis. Best Pract Res Clin Rheumatol 2018;32(1):31–51.
47. Hoffman GS, Kerr GS, Leavitt RY, et al. Wegener granulomatosis: an analysis of 158 patients. Ann Intern Med 1992;116(6):488–98.
48. Jones RB, Tervaert JWC, Hauser T, et al. Rituximab versus cyclophosphamide in ANCA-associated renal vasculitis. N Engl J Med 2010;363(3):211–20.
49. Stone JH, Merkel PA, Spiera R, et al. Rituximab versus cyclophosphamide for ANCA-associated vasculitis. N Engl J Med 2010;363(3):221–32.

Renovascular Hypertension

Sai Sudha Mannemuddhu, MD[a], Jason C. Ojeda, MD[b],
Anju Yadav, MD[c],*

KEYWORDS

- Resistant hypertension • Renovascular hypertension • Secondary hypertension
- Renal artery stenosis • Fibromuscular dysplasia • Renal vascular angioplasty

KEY POINTS

- Renovascular hypertension is one of the common causes of secondary hypertension which remains underdiagnosed.
- Patients usually present with suboptimal blood pressure control despite being on multiple antihypertensives.
- High index of suspicion along with prompt evaluation and management can potentially prevent end-organ damage.
- Pharmacologic and life style modifications play a major role in the management of hypertension, but some patients may benefit from timely surgical intervention. Careful patient selection is the key.

Case 1: A 19-year-old man presents to the clinic with new-onset hypertension (HTN). He has elevated blood pressures (BPs) in both his arms. There was no radio-radial or radio-femoral delay. His urinalysis showed 2+ protein with first morning urine protein creatinine ratio of 0.7 mg/g. His basal metabolic panel (BMP) showed serum creatinine (S. Cr) of 0.5 mg/dL with estimated glomerular filtration rate (eGFR) of 130 mL/min. His electrocardiogram (EKG) and transthoracic echocardiogram (ECHO) were normal. He was started on Lisinopril 20 mg daily and BMP was repeated in a week that showed elevated S. Cr of 1 mg/dL. What is the next step?

Case 2: A 28-year-old woman was found to have elevated BP during multiple physician visits. No family history (hx) of HTN. Her history is significant for ovarian cancer that was treated with radiation approximately 8 years ago. BPs were repeatedly elevated on both upper extremities. There was no radio-radial or radio-femoral delay.

[a] Department of Pediatrics, Division of Nephrology, University of Florida-College of Medicine, 1600 Southwest Archer Road, HD-214, Gainesville, FL 32610, USA; [b] Department of Internal Medicine, Thomas Jefferson University, 833 Chestnut Street, Suite 701, Philadelphia, PA 19107, USA; [c] Division of Nephrology, Hypertension and Transplantation, Thomas Jefferson University, 833 Chestnut Street, Suite 700, Philadelphia, PA 19107, USA
* Corresponding author.
E-mail address: anju.yadav@jefferson.edu
Twitter: @drM_sudha (S.S.M.); @docanjuyadav (A.Y.)

Prim Care Clin Office Pract 47 (2020) 631–644
https://doi.org/10.1016/j.pop.2020.08.009
0095-4543/20/© 2020 Elsevier Inc. All rights reserved.

Her physical examination was unremarkable with no renal masses, and no carotid, renal, or femoral artery bruits. Her fundus eye examination was normal. Her BMP, urinalysis, complete blood count, erythrocyte sedimentation rate, and liver function tests were all normal. Her EKG and ECHO were unremarkable. What is the next step in management?

Case 3: A 54-year-old man with diabetes mellitus (DM), HTN, and coronary artery disease (CAD) presents to the office for follow-up after a visit to the emergency room for nephrolithiasis. His pain has resolved, and he passed the 3-mm stone without complication, but in the workup of his pain, he had a renal ultrasound that showed evidence of 2-cm discrepancy in the kidney size. He feels well and his BP is 126/74 mm Hg. He is on metformin, lisinopril, metoprolol, aspirin, and clopidogrel, which he tolerates well. His creatinine is 1.0 mg/dL and his HbA1C is 6.8%. He follows up regularly and reports no symptoms of dyspnea. What is your next step in management? Lets see if we can find answers to these.

INTRODUCTION

When a patient presents to the office with difficult to control or resistant HTN, a workup for secondary causes of HTN is warranted. Renovascular hypertension (RVH) is an important consideration in such circumstances. Before delving into the details of RVH, it is important to establish a few definitions.

HTN is defined as systolic BP (SBP) $\geq$130 mm Hg and diastolic blood pressure (DBP) $\geq$80 mm Hg using a manual blood pressure monitor (American Heart Association [AHA] guidelines[1]). AHA and International Society of Hypertension (ISH)[2] guidelines for hypertension classification are as follows.

AHA guidelines (BP represented as SBP/DBP in mm Hg. *Normal: <120/and <80, Elevated BP: 120–129/and <80, Stage I HTN: 130–139/or 80–89, Stage II HTN: $\geq$140/or >90).*

ISH Guidelines *(Normal: <130/and <85, High Normal BP: 130–139/and/or 85–89, Stage I HTN: 140–159/and/or 89–99, Stage II HTN: $\geq$160/and/or $\geq$100).*

Ambulatory BP monitoring (ABPM) is the gold standard in diagnosing hypertension. ISH guidelines recommend following values for the diagnosis of HTN. *Office BP ($\geq$140 and/or $\geq$90); Average ABPM (24-h: $\geq$130 and/or $\geq$80, Daytime or awake: $\geq$135 and/or $\geq$85, Nighttime/Asleep: $\geq$120 and/or $\geq$70); Home BP measurement (HBPM): $\geq$135 and/or $\geq$85.*

What Is the Correct Way of Checking BP?

All patients should be instructed to check BP appropriately at home. AHA BP measurement instructions:

- Check BP in a calm environment, seated on a chair for at least 5 minutes, with arms resting on side, legs uncrossed with feet on floor, and back supported.
- At least 2 readings 5-10 minutes apart in the morning before medications, and in the evening before dinner are required.
- Using a properly calibrated machine with appropriate size arm cuff with monitor placed at the level of the heart is very important.
- At the time of BP measurement, ensure that there was no smoking, exercise, or consumption of caffeinated drinks or alcohol within 30 minutes of measurement and that the bladder should be empty.

Resistant hypertension (RH): RH is defined as uncontrolled BP $\geq$130/80 mm Hg, despite concurrent use of 3 appropriate antihypertensive medications (angiotensin-converting enzyme [ACE] inhibitors/aldosterone receptor blocker (ARB) plus a calcium channel blocker (CCB) in appropriate doses including a diuretic.[3] The National Health and Nutrition Examination Survey (NHANES) data study showed that RH had a prevalence of 20.7% during 2005 to 2008.[4] *Pseudo-RH* is a term used when BPs are elevated due to white coat effect, insufficient drug therapy, failure to adhere to lifestyle modifications, nonadherence to medication, poor measurement technique, or use of medications/substances that interfere with blood pressure.[5]

Refractory HTN (RFH): RFH is a subset of RH that is defined as failure to achieve target BP despite 5 or more anti-HTN drugs, which includes a diuretic.[6] ALLHAT (antihypertensive and lipid lowering treatment to prevent heart attack trial) data showed that 12.7% had treatment-resistant HTN.[7] RFH is found to be common in African American individuals, women, and patients with chronic kidney disease with creatinine greater than 1.5 mg/dL, high body mass index, or DM.[7]

Secondary HTN: Secondary hypertension, accounting for ~10% of all hypertension, refers to HTN with a specific and often a remediable cause[8] (**Box 1**).

In this article, discussion focuses mainly on renovascular hypertension, the most common cause of secondary HTN.[9]

RENOVASCULAR HYPERTENSION

RVH is a rise in arterial pressure attributable to decreased kidney perfusion.[10] Although RVH can be an asymptomatic and incidental finding, it can have long-term negative consequences, including ischemic nephropathy, cardiovascular disease, congestive heart failure, and stroke. Due to insensitivity of diagnostic testing and the lack of compelling data for benefits associated with interventions, particularly in patients with uncomplicated HTN, it is advisable to be careful regarding workup for RVH. It should be pursued in patients with high likelihood of the disease. With an aging population with multiple comorbidities, the incidence of cardiovascular events and deaths have increased in patients older than 67 years, and have an increasing incidence of new diagnosis of RVH on Medicare records.[11] It is important to recognize patients who may benefit from diagnosis and intervention for RVH.

INCIDENCE AND PREVALENCE

RVH is a heterogeneous condition with multiple possible etiologies, as outlined in **Box 2**. RVH accounts for 1% to 5% of the general hypertensive population and

---

Box 1
Most common secondary causes of hypertension (HTN)

- Renal parenchymal disease/chronic kidney disease
- Renovascular HTN (most common)
- Adrenal disorders: primary hyperaldosteronism, Cushing syndrome
- Pheochromocytoma
- Thyroid disorders
- Coarctation of the aorta
- Obstructive sleep apnea
- Medication-induced HTN
- Intracranial tumor

> **Box 2**
> **Causes of renovascular hypertension (RVH)**
>
> Renal artery stenosis (RAS)
>
> Atherosclerotic renal artery disease (ARAD) or fibromuscular dysplasia (FMD)
>
> Systemic vasculitis
>
> Renal arterial aneurysm
>
> Arteriovenous fistula
>
> Aortic or renal artery dissection
>
> Systemic emboli generated during endovascular manipulation
>
> Renin-secreting renal tumor
>
> Extrinsic compression of either kidney or renal artery due to tumors or metastasis
>
> Subcapsular intrarenal hematoma
>
> Radiation fibrosis
>
> *Data from* Puar THK, Mok Y, Debajyoti R, et al. Secondary hypertension in adults. Singapore Med. J. 2016;57(5):228–32; and Badila E, Tintea E. How to manage renovascular hypertension. e-Journal of Cardiology Practice 2014;13:8–9.

constitutes approximately 20% to 40% of the cases of secondary HTN.[12,13] A prospective study in 96 young patients identified secondary hypertension in 18.1%, with RVH accounting for 75% cases.[14] Epidemiologic studies have established a strong association between atherosclerotic renal artery disease (ARAD) and cardiovascular risk. There is an epidemiologic suggestion that individuals with refractory heart failure and end-stage kidney disease (ESKD) may have demonstrable ARAD in 40% to 50% of cases.[10]

Renal artery stenosis (RAS): RAS is one of the important causes of RVH and an underrecognized cause of ESKD. It is caused predominantly by atherosclerotic disease (~90%) and by fibromuscular dysplasia[15] (**Fig. 1**).

Atherosclerotic renal artery disease (ARAD): Patients are usually older than 50 years, with associated comorbid conditions like HTN, smoking, and DM. It usually affects ostium and the proximal one-third of the renal artery's branch. The true prevalence is unknown and likely underestimated, as not all patients present clinically. ARAD has become the leading cause of ESKD in elderly individuals.[15] This is associated

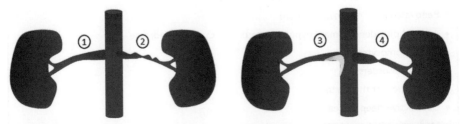

Fig. 1. Common causes of RAS. Normal renal artery (1), Fibromuscular dysplasia (2), Atherosclerotic RAS (3), and narrowing of the artery (4). (*Courtesy of* Sai Sudha Mannemuddhu, MD, FAAP, Knoxville, TN.)

with accelerated and more severe target organ injury than seen with essential HTN.[16] Caps and colleagues[17] showed that cumulative incidence of renal atrophy (>1 cm loss in renal length) at 2 years was 5.5%, 11.7%, and 20.8%, when baseline RAS was none, less than 60%, and 60%, respectively. Other studies showed that total occlusion occurred in 7% to 16% of patients in 1 to 2 years.[18,19]

Fibromuscular dysplasia (FMD) is a noninflammatory, nonatherosclerotic vascular disease (medial fibroplasia) that affects small to medium-sized arteries like renal vessels (60%–75%) and are located in the distal two-thirds of the renal arteries, their secondary or distal branches. It accounts for 10% to 20% of documented patients with RAS and occurs mostly in women 15 to 50 years of age.[15]

ARAD can be differentiated from FMD based on the affected site radiological studies, as mentioned previously.[20] This distinction is important, and a high index of suspicion is necessary, as early diagnosis and prompt treatment can potentially result in rapid and complete recovery in FMD. Unlike ARAD, FMD rarely leads to ESKD and/ or flash pulmonary edema. Polyarteritis nodosa with multiple aneurysms can mimic FMD, so careful consideration is warranted.

PATHOGENESIS/PATHOPHYSIOLOGY

In the mid-twentieth century, Goldblatt kidney models demonstrated for the first time that the renin-angiotensin-aldosterone-system (RAAS) activation and sodium retention play a major role in experimental RVH.[21–23] As depicted in **Fig. 2**A, 2-kidney 1-clip Goldblatt hypertension model, the ischemic kidney secretes renin, which leads to increased angiotensin II and aldosterone, resulting in vasoconstriction and water and sodium retention, respectively (angiotensin-dependent HTN). Elevated BP leads to pressure natriuresis via the normal kidney and therefore, there is no sodium retention. Though volume status is optimized, this is often insufficient to control BP.

In 1-kidney 1-clip or 2-kidney 2-clip Goldblatt hypertension models, both the kidneys or the solitary kidney artery are occluded. There is no normal kidney to compensate, leading to volume-dependent HTN and suppression of renin secretion (**Fig. 2**B).

Decreased blood flow to kidney parenchyma leads to RAAS activation, which causes RVH. Prolonged activation of RAAS leads to sympathetic nervous system activation, decreased nitric oxide and prostacyclin synthesis, and increased profibrotic growth factors. This causes cardiac and vascular remodeling, and ischemic kidney damage leading to nephrosclerosis[15] (**Fig. 3**).

CLINICAL PRESENTATION

RVH can present with a spectrum of progressive clinical manifestations ranging from minor degrees of HTN to ischemic nephropathy.[9,24,25] **Box 3** enumerates clinical and investigational clues to the diagnosis of RVH.

Outpatient Workup

Once secondary hypertension is suspected to be due to renovascular hypertension, a series of laboratory and imaging studies are indicated for confirmation. See **Box 4**.

Imaging

Duplex ultrasonography: Classically, RAS is diagnosed when a renal artery Doppler ultrasound shows more than 75% narrowing of the diameter of the main renal artery, or greater than 50% luminal narrowing with a post stenotic dilatation. A duplex scan correlates well with contrast-enhanced angiography. This study should ideally be performed at a center where such ultrasound imaging is done in high volume, as it

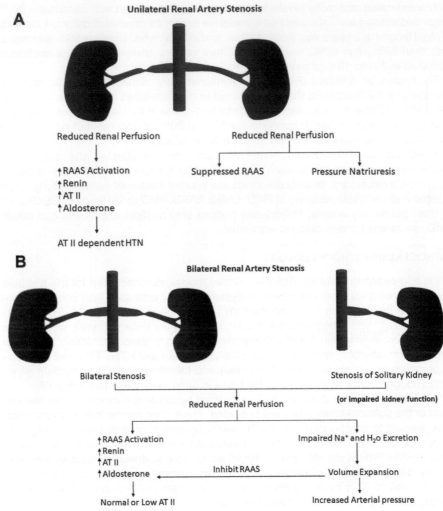

Fig. 2. Goldblatt kidney model depicting pathophysiology of RVH. (*A*) Two-kidney 1-clip Goldblatt hypertension. (*B*) One-clip 1-kidney or 2-kidney 2-clip Goldblatt hypertension. AT II, Angiotensin II (*Adapted from* Herrmann SM, Textor SC. Syndromes of renovascular hypertension. In: Singh SK, Agarwal R, editors. Core concepts in hypertension in kidney disease. New York: Springer; 2016. p. 63–83; with permission.)

requires a high technical expertise in performing and analyzing. However, failure rate of detection is 10% to 20% in the presence of obesity or bowel gas, as it is highly operator dependent, and due to the possibility of a stenotic accessory artery, which cannot be excluded[20] (**Fig. 4**A).

Nuclear medicine ACE inhibitor renography: Captopril renography (DTPA renography) is a safe noninvasive tool used in the screening for RAS. Sensitivity and specificity decrease in the presence of decreased kidney function. This is not a preferred or first choice for screening.

Computed tomography (CT) and MR angiography (CTA and MRA): It is the most specific tool in diagnosis with comparable sensitivity and specificity. MRA has an additional advantage of not having radiation exposure and limited nephrotoxicity.

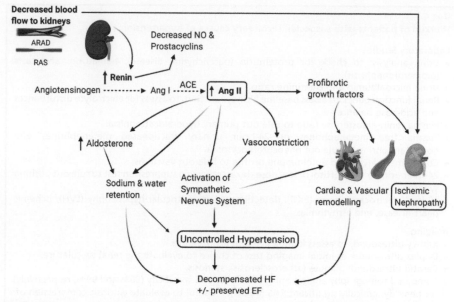

Fig. 3. Consequences and complications of RAS. AT II, Angiotensin II; EF, ejection fraction; H_2O, water; HF, heart failure; HTN, hypertension; Na, Sodium; NO, nitric oxide. (*Courtesy of* Sai Sudha Mannemuddhu, MD, FAAP, Knoxville, TN.)

Box 3
Clinical, laboratory, and imaging features of RVH

History and physical examination clues:
- Early age of onset of HTN less than 30 years (consider FMD) or later in life greater than 50 years (consider ARAD)
- Worsening of previously well controlled HTN.
- Resistant HTN.
- History of multiple admissions to hospitals with hypertensive crisis, flash pulmonary edema.
- History of atherosclerotic diseases such as carotid artery stenosis, peripheral artery stenosis, or coronary artery disease (CAD).
- Angina without significant CAD in hypertensive patients.
- A premenopausal female patient (15–50 years) with HTN is most likely to have FMD.
- Accelerated or malignant hypertension or refractory HTN or resistant hypertension with 3 antihypertensives including a diuretic.

Laboratory and imaging studies
- Unilateral small kidney; difference in two kidney size greater than 1.5 cm in length on renal ultrasound.
- Rapid elevation in creatinine after angiotensin-converting enzyme inhibitors (ACE-I) or aldosterone receptor blockers are initiated.
- Recurrent flash pulmonary edema, Congestive heart failure (CHF) in a hypertensive patient, especially in heart failure with preserved ejection fraction.
- Keith-Wegener-Barker grade III or IV fundi on retinal examination.
- ARAD or atherosclerotic lesions in nonrenal vasculature in patient with HTN.
- Unexplained hypokalemia and metabolic alkalosis.
- Ankle-brachial index: peripheral (lower extremity) artery disease.

Box 4
Workup of patients with suspected secondary causes of hypertension

Laboratory Studies
- Urine analysis: to check for proteinuria (parenchymal disease), hematuria, and casts (glomerulonephritis).
- Urine microalbumin and creatinine ratio.
- Renal function panel: to assess baseline kidney function, to assess for electrolyte disturbances and acid-base balance.
- Plasma renin-aldosterone ratio to rule out primary hyperaldosteronism.
- Plasma free metanephrines or 24-hour urinary fractionated metanephrines and normetanephrine to rule out pheochromocytoma.
- Complement levels and autoimmune profile to rule out vasculitis.
- 24-hour urinary free cortisol or low dose dexamethasone suppression test to rule out Cushing syndrome.
- 12-lead electrocardiogram (EKG): detection of left ventricular hypertrophy (LVH), ischemic heart disease, and arrhythmias.

Imaging
- Kidney ultrasound: to assess kidney size and echotexture.
- Duplex ultrasound: as initial imaging test of choice to evaluate the renal vasculature.
- Carotid ultrasound: plaques (atherosclerosis), stenosis.
- Computed tomography angiography: sensitivity and specificity (96% and 99%, respectively) for hemodynamically significant RAS (>50%).[13] Useful to evaluate extrinsic compression of renal arteries, FMD, arterial dissection, and surrounding structures.
- MR angiography: sensitivity and specificity (97% and 92%, respectively) in detecting RAS; however it can overestimate stenosis.
- Nuclear medicine ACE-I renography: variable sensitivity (74%–94%) and specificity (59%–95%).[26]
- Catheter angiography and digital subtraction angiography (DSA): gold standard.
- Echocardiography (ECHO): Helpful in the detection of LVH, structural heart disease, coarctation of aorta, systolic and diastolic function, ischemic heart disease.

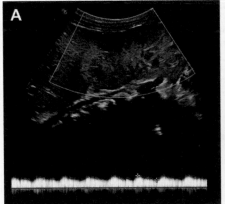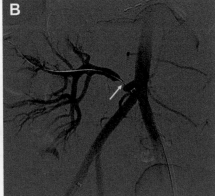

Fig. 4. Doppler sonogram and catheter angiogram showing RAS. (*A*) Doppler sonogram of kidneys showing decreased blood flow and pulsus parvus tardus. (*B*) Conventional catheter angiogram showing RAS. Arrow indicating proximal arterial lumen narrowing. (*Courtesy of Sai Sudha Mannemuddhu, MD, FAAP, Knoxville, TN.*)

Catheter angiography: This is the gold standard in diagnosing renal artery FMD (**Fig. 4**B). Digital subtraction angiography *(DSA)* is intra-arterial angiogram with digital subtraction. It is most useful in patients with a high index of suspicion with negative or disparity between imaging findings and in whom intervention is anticipated. Indications are FMD ("string of beads" appearance),[15] short duration of BP elevation before diagnosis of RAS and recurrent flash pulmonary edema.

Echocardiogram: Physicians should be alerted to look for RAS when a patient presents with heart failure out of proportion to left ventricular dysfunction.[15]

DIFFERENTIAL DIAGNOSIS

The differential diagnosis for renovascular hypertension is vast and therefore, a complete and thoughtful history must be taken including asking related symptom questions as well as obtaining a comprehensive list of medications including over-the-counter medications. See **Box 5**.

Box 5
Differential diagnosis of RVH[2,27]

- *Pheochromocytoma*: flushing, headache, tachycardia, and episodic uncontrolled hypertension.

- *Primary hyperaldosteronism*: persistent hypokalemia and metabolic alkalosis.

- *Cushing syndrome*: moon facies, buffalo hump, proximal myopathy, glucose intolerance, abdominal striae, and central obesity.

- *Thyroid disorders*: skin changes, weight changes, cold/heat intolerance, palpitations, and mood disturbances. Free T4 and thyroid-stimulating hormone aids in diagnosis.

- *Obstructive sleep apnea*: obesity with increased neck circumference and history of snoring; polysomnography is diagnostic.

- *Coarctation of the aorta:* systolic murmur, radio-femoral delay, and upper extremity hypertension. Diagnosed with MRA or CTA.

- *Medication-induced HTN*: medications causing or interfering with treatment of HTN.
  - Oral contraceptives: increases with high doses of estrogen.
  - Steroids.
  - Nonsteroidal anti-inflammatory drugs (NSAIDs): celecoxib and nonselective NSAIDs can increase blood pressure, but no increase in blood pressure is observed with aspirin. NSAIDs can antagonize the effects of renin-angiotensin-aldosterone-system inhibitors and beta blockers.
  - Acetaminophen: Daily use can increase relative of HTN.
  - Antidepressants: selective norepinephrine and serotonin reuptake inhibitors and tricyclic antidepressants can cause increased blood pressure. No increases in blood pressure with selective serotonin reuptake inhibitors.
  - Sympathomimetics (amphetamines, decongestants, diet pills).
  - Illicit drugs and other herbal preparations: cocaine, alcohol, ma-huang, ginseng at high doses, licorice, St. John's wort, yohimbine.
  - Others are antimigraine serotonergics, recombinant human erythropoietin, calcineurin inhibitors, antiangiogenesis and kinase inhibitors, 11 ß-hydroxysteroid dehydrogenase type 2 inhibitors.

Data from Unger T, Borghi C, Charchar F, et al. 2020 International Society of Hypertension global hypertension practice guidelines. Hypertension. 2020;75(6):1334–57; with permission; and Puar THK, Mok Y, Debajyoti R, et al. Secondary hypertension in adults. Singapore Med. J. 2016;57(5):228–32.

MANAGEMENT
Lifestyle Modifications

Lifestyle modifications like smoking cessation, low-salt diet, regular exercise, and optimal weight management play a significant role in the control of HTN and thus preventing potentially associated negative effects of RVH on cardiovascular and renal function.

Medical Management

- *Hypertension*: BP target for the general population is BP ≤140/90 mm Hg; For those populations with comorbidities like diabetes, heart disease, kidney disease, or proteinuria BP target is lower ≤130/80 mm Hg. RAAS blockade is the first-line agent.[2]
- *Dyslipidemia*: target low-density lipoprotein level is <100 mg/dL; a level of less than 70 mg/dL is desired particularly in patients with comorbidities.
- *Diabetes*: target HbA1C <7 g/dL.
- *Anti-platelet agents* such as aspirin, clopidogrel, or ticlopidine are recommended.
- Chronic kidney disease management—electrolyte, anemia, and bone mineral disease management

Surgical Management

Percutaneous angioplasty is the treatment of choice for renovascular hypertension due to FMD and for patients with atherosclerotic RAS that is not controlled with medications.[28]

The American College of Cardiology (ACC)/AHA guidelines recommend revascularization for renal artery disease in the following scenarios:

1. Patients with hemodynamically significant RAS and recurrent, unexplained congestive heart failure or sudden, unexplained pulmonary edema (Class Ia)
2. Hemodynamically significant RAS and accelerated hypertension, RH, malignant hypertension or hypertension with an unexplained unilateral small kidney, and hypertension with intolerance to medication (Class IIa)
3. Patients with bilateral RAS and progressive chronic kidney disease or a RAS to a solitary functioning kidney (Class IIa)
4. Patients with hemodynamically significant RAS and unstable angina (Class IIa)
5. Asymptomatic bilateral or solitary viable kidney with hemodynamically significant RAS (Class IIb)
6. Patients with RAS and chronic renal insufficiency with unilateral RAS (Class IIb)
7. In addition to angioplasty, renal stent placement is indicated for patients with ostial atherosclerotic lesions (Class I)

All the trials studying the effect of renal artery angioplasty and stenting trials have consistently failed to show benefit with renal artery stenting compared with medical treatment, in terms of patient survival, cardiovascular events, renal function, or blood pressure (**Table 1**). Several significant side effects associated with these interventions were noted in all these trials including death and toe of limb amputation.

A meta-analysis of 7 trials by Zhu and colleagues[31] revealed that medical management is as effective as percutaneous revascularization in the treatment of RAS.

Another meta-analysis by Nordmann and colleagues[32] showed that there are only 3 randomized trials (a total of 210 patients) comparing medical management with balloon angioplasty prospectively. Balloon angioplasty showed modest effect in

Table 1
Randomized controlled trials comparing medical management with percutaneous revascularization

Trial	Criteria	n	Follow-up	Primary Endpoint	Results
STAR Trial[29]	RAS (>50% stenosis)	140	2 y	>20% decrease in Cr clearance	No significant difference in renal function, BP, cardiovascular mortality, and morbidity
ASTRAL Trial[30]	RAS (unilateral or bilateral)	806	34 mo	Change in renal function	No significant difference in renal function, BP, cardiovascular events, and mortality
CORAL trial[12]	RAS (stenosis >80% or >60% stenosis with an SBP gradient >20 mm Hg)	947	43 mo	Composite of death from cardiovascular or renal causes, stroke, MI, CHF hospitalization, renal insufficiency, or permanent RRT	No significant difference in the occurrence of primary composite endpoint, any of the individual components of the composite endpoints, or all-cause mortality

Abbreviations: BP, blood pressure; CHF, congestive heart failure; Cr, creatinine; MI, myocardial infarction; RAS, renal artery stenosis; RRT, renal replacement therapy; SBP, systolic BP.

reducing BPs in patients with RAS but no evidence supporting its use in improving or preserving renal function.

In a selective patient population renal vascularization is beneficial. Careful selection should be carried out with a multidisciplinary approach and informed decision making in such cases. Factors that can predict the outcome of percutaneous procedure are listed in **Table 2**.

The goal of surgical revascularization is correction of RVH with preservation of renal function. In a person with failed angioplasty with/without stenting and suboptimal management with medical therapy, surgical interventions can be considered, like auto transplantation, and aortorenal and aorto-aortic bypass. In selected refractory cases, nephrectomy can be considered as well.

Nephrology consultation/referral to evaluate renovascular hypertension (ACC/AHA guidelines)

1. Acute rise in BP in a patient with previously stable readings or worsening of previously controlled HTN
2. Accelerated or malignant or refractory HTN
3. When history, examination, and initial screening test suggest secondary causes of RH

Table 2
Factors predicting probable benefit from invasive therapy of renovascular hypertension[9,33]

	Probable Benefit	Probable Not Benefit
Hx of HTN	<10 y	>10 y
Refractory HTN	Present	Absent
Hx of Cholesterol Embolization	Absent	Present
Kidney Function	Deteriorating	Stable
Proteinuria	<1 g/d	>1 g/d
Renal artery stenosis	<70%	≥70%
Renal resistive index	<80 mm Hg	≥80 mm Hg
Unilateral small kidney (<7.5 cm)	Absent	Present
Flash pulmonary edema	Present	Absent

Abbreviations: HTN, hypertension; Hx, history.
Data from Badila E, Tintea E. How to manage renovascular hypertension. e-Journal of Cardiology Practice 2014;13:8–9; and Feldman L, Beberashvili I, Averbukh Z, et al. Renal artery stenosis of solitary kidney: the dilemma. Ren. Fail. 2004;26:525–9.

4. Discrepancy in kidney size (>1.5 cm) on imaging or decreased blood flow on Doppler
5. Evidence of target organ damage or clinical manifestations of cardiovascular disease
6. Greater than 30% rise in creatinine after initiation of ACE inhibitor or ARB or presentation suggestive of flash pulmonary edema
7. Consideration of device therapy to control blood pressure when all drug interventions have been exhausted
8. Young hypertensive patients (<40 years of age)

ANSWERS TO THE CASES

1. Most likely cause is RVH and the first line of investigation would be Doppler renal ultrasound.
2. Fibromuscular dysplasia of the left renal artery is the likely diagnosis. Radionuclide scan of the kidney followed by arterial renogram for the diagnosis.
3. Although this patient would benefit from referral to nephrology and close monitoring in primary care, he is currently optimized with medical therapy and likely would not benefit from a workup for RVH at this time. He likely does have ARAD but would not be a candidate for intervention beyond his current medical regimen due to ischemic kidney and stable renal function with good BP control. Maximize and optimize medical therapy.

SUMMARY

RVH accounts for 1% to 5% of the general hypertensive population and constitutes approximately 20% to 40% of the cases of secondary HTN. Therefore, it is important to distinguish and recognize the symptoms and signs of RVH to aid with early diagnosis and referral, which is vital for timely management, and to prevent end-organ damage. Differentiating ARAD versus FMD is critical when evaluating RVH because the line of management differs. Lifestyle modifications and pharmacologic measures play a very important role in management. Pharmacologic therapy should be optimized before considering surgical management. In selected cases, angioplasty with stenting can be considered; however, outcome of these interventions depends on expertise and patient selection. With meticulous approach and timely diagnosis, the ill effects of renovascular hypertension can be managed effectively and sometimes completely reversed.

ACKNOWLEDGMENTS

The authors thank Matthew Sparks MD, FASN, FAHA for his continued support and assistance with this article.

DISCLOSURE

The authors have nothing to disclose.

REFERENCES

1. Flack JM, Calhoun D, Schiffrin EL. The New ACC/AHA Hypertension Guidelines for the Prevention, Detection, Evaluation, and Management of High Blood Pressure in Adults. Am J Hypertens 2018;31(2):133–5.
2. Unger T, Borghi C, Charchar F, et al. 2020 International Society of Hypertension Global Hypertension Practice Guidelines. Hypertension 2020;75(6):1334–57.
3. Reboussin DM, Allen NB, Griswold ME, et al. Systematic Review for the 2017 ACC/AHA/AAPA/ABC/ACPM/AGS/APhA/ASH/ASPC/NMA/PCNA Guideline for the Prevention, Detection, Evaluation, and Management of High Blood Pressure in Adults: A Report of the American College of Cardiology/American Heart Association Task Force on Clinical Practice Guidelines. Hypertension 2018;71: e116–35.
4. Roberie DR, Elliott WJ. What is the prevalence of resistant hypertension in the United States? Curr Opin Cardiol 2012;27(4):386–91.
5. Yaxley JP, Thambar SV. Resistant hypertension: an approach to management in primary care. J Fam Med Prim Care 2015;4(2):193–9.
6. Acelajado MC, Pisoni R, Dudenbostel T, et al. Refractory hypertension: definition, prevalence, and patient characteristics. J Clin Hypertens (Greenwich) 2012; 14(1):7–12.
7. Muntner P, Davis BR, Cushman WC, et al. Treatment-resistant hypertension and the incidence of cardiovascular disease and end-stage renal disease: results from the Antihypertensive and Lipid-Lowering Treatment to Prevent Heart Attack Trial (ALLHAT). Hypertension 2014;64(5):1012–21.
8. Puar TH, Mok Y, Debajyoti R, et al. Secondary hypertension in adults. Singapore Med J 2016;57(5):228–32.
9. Badila E, Tintea E. How to manage renovascular hypertension. J Cardiol Pract 2014;13:8–9.
10. Textor SC, Lerman L. Renovascular hypertension and ischemic nephropathy. Am J Hypertens 2010;23(11):1159–69.
11. Kalra PA, Guo H, Kausz AT, et al. Atherosclerotic renovascular disease in United States patients aged 67 years or older: Risk factors, revascularization, and prognosis. Kidney Int 2005;68(1):293–301.
12. Cooper CJ, Murphy TP, Cutlip DE, et al. Stenting and medical therapy for atherosclerotic renal-artery stenosis. N Engl J Med 2014;370(1):13–22.
13. Rountas C, Vlychou M, Vassiou K, et al. Imaging modalities for renal artery stenosis in suspected renovascular hypertension: prospective intraindividual comparison of color Doppler US, CT angiography, GD-enhanced MR angiography, and digital subtraction angiography. Ren Fail 2007;29(3):295–302.

14. Little MA, O'Brien E, Owens P, et al. A longitudinal study of the yield and clinical utility of a specifically designed secondary hypertension investigation protocol. Ren Fail 2003;25(5):709–17.
15. Fernando D, Garasic J. Percutaneous intervention for renovascular disease: rationale and patient selection. Curr Opin Cardiol 2004;19(6):582–8.
16. Textor SC. Current approaches to renovascular hypertension. Med Clin North Am 2009;93(3):717–32.
17. Caps MT, Zierler RE, Polissar NL, et al. Risk of atrophy in kidneys with atherosclerotic renal artery stenosis. Kidney Int 1998;53(3):735–42.
18. Zierler RE, Bergelin RO, Davidson RC, et al. A prospective study of disease progression in patients with atherosclerotic renal artery stenosis. Am J Hypertens 1996;9(11):1055–61.
19. Harden PN, MacLeod MJ, Rodger RS, et al. Effect of renal-artery stenting on progression of renovascular renal failure. Lancet 1997;349(9059):1133–6.
20. Ralapanawa DMPUK, Jayawickreme KP, Ekanayake EMM. A case of treatable hypertension: fibromuscular dysplasia of renal arteries. BMC Res Notes 2016;9:6.
21. Pickering TG. Renovascular hypertension: etiology and pathophysiology. Semin Nucl Med 1989;19(2):79–88.
22. Van Epps HL. Harry Goldblatt and the discovery of renin. J Exp Med 2005;201(9): 1351.
23. Herrmann SM, Textor SC. Syndromes of renovascular hypertension. In: Singh AK, Agarwal R, editors. Core concepts in hypertension in kidney disease. New York: Springer; 2016. p. 63–83.
24. Textor SC. Renal arterial disease and hypertension. Med Clin North Am 2017; 101(1):65–79.
25. Nair R, Vaqar S. Renovascular Hypertension. [Updated 2020 May 30]. In: StatPearls [Internet]. Treasure Island (FL): StatPearls Publishing; 2020 Jan-. Available at: https://www.ncbi.nlm.nih.gov/books/NBK551587/
26. Huot SJ, Hansson JH, Dey H, et al. Utility of captopril renal scans for detecting renal artery stenosis. Arch Intern Med 2002;162(17):1981–4.
27. Puar TH, Mok Y, Debajyoti R, et al. Secondary hypertension in adults. Singapore Med J 2016;57(5):228–32.
28. Chrysant SG, Chrysant GS. Treatment of hypertension in patients with renal artery stenosis due to fibromuscular dysplasia of the renal arteries. Cardiovasc Diagn Ther 2014;4(1):36–43.
29. Bax L, Woittiez AJ, Kouwenberg HJ, et al. Stent placement in patients with atherosclerotic renal artery stenosis and impaired renal function: a randomized trial. Ann Intern Med 2009;150:840–8. W150–1.
30. ASTRAL Investigators, Wheatley K, Ives N, Gray R, et al. Revascularization versus medical therapy for renal-artery stenosis. N Engl J Med 2009;361: 1953–62.
31. Zhu Y, Ren J, Ma X, et al. Percutaneous revascularization for atherosclerotic renal artery stenosis: a meta-analysis of randomized controlled trials. Ann Vasc Surg 2015;29(7):1457–67.
32. Nordmann AJ, Woo K, Parkes R, et al. Balloon angioplasty or medical therapy for hypertensive patients with atherosclerotic renal artery stenosis? A meta-analysis of randomized controlled trials. Am J Med 2003;114(1):44–50.
33. Feldman L, Beberashvili I, Averbukh Z, et al. Renal artery stenosis of solitary kidney: the dilemma. Ren Fail 2004;26(5):525–9.

Diabetic Kidney Disease

Ryan Bonner, MD, Oltjon Albajrami, MD, James Hudspeth, MD,
Ashish Upadhyay, MD*

KEYWORDS

- Diabetic kidney disease • Diabetic nephropathy • Chronic kidney disease
- Albuminuria

KEY POINTS

- Diabetic kidney disease (DKD) is the most common cause of chronic kidney disease in the United States and affects 30% to 40% of patients with diabetes mellitus.
- The progression of DKD is characterized by a decline in kidney function and worsening albuminuria and is associated with increased cardiovascular and all-cause mortality.
- Mainstays of management of DKD continue to be effective glycemic and blood pressure control and blockade of the renin-angiotensin-aldosterone system.
- Emerging therapies, such as sodium-glucose cotransporter 2 inhibitors and glucagon-like peptide-1 analogues, in the right setting, can play an important role in slowing DKD progression.

EPIDEMIOLOGY

Chronic kidney disease (CKD) affects a 15% of Americans, and diabetic kidney disease (DKD) is the most common cause of kidney failure.[1,2] Although the incidence of diabetes-related kidney failure has slowed over the past 2 decades, approximately 30% of patients with type 1 diabetes mellitus (T1DM) and 40% of patients with type 2 diabetes mellitus (T2DM) develop some form of CKD.[1] Because mortality and morbidity risks rise with CKD progression, it is imperative to prioritize prevention, recognition, and management of DKD in the primary care setting.[3]

PATHOGENESIS/PATHOPHYSIOLOGY

DKD is driven primarily by 3 intersecting processes: hyperfiltration injury to the glomerular filtration barrier (GFB), expansion of the glomerular mesangium, and oxidative stress. Development of these processes is multifactorial and thought to be related to hemodynamic, metabolic, and immune pathology, which are discussed individually and summarized in **Fig. 1.**

Section of Nephrology, Department of Medicine, Boston Medical Center and Boston University School of Medicine, 800 Harrison Avenue, G009, Boston, MA 02118, USA
* Corresponding author.
E-mail address: Ashish.Upadhyay@bmc.org

Prim Care Clin Office Pract 47 (2020) 645–659
https://doi.org/10.1016/j.pop.2020.08.004
0095-4543/20/© 2020 Elsevier Inc. All rights reserved.

primarycare.theclinics.com

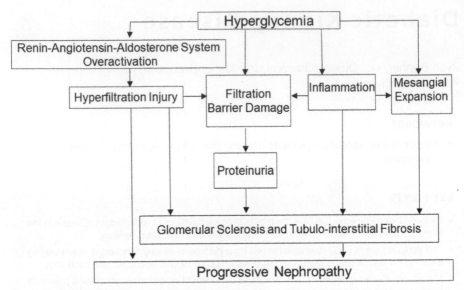

Fig. 1. Pathophysiology of diabetic kidney disease.

Hemodynamic Alterations

Aberrant activation of the renin-angiotensin-aldosterone system (RAAS) is known to cause vasoconstriction of the efferent arteriole, leading to an increase in intraglomerular pressure. High intraglomerular pressure and the resultant hyperfiltration injury of the GFB, over time, manifest as albuminuria and lower glomerular filtration rate (GFR). Additionally, excess endothelin-1 activity causes vasoconstriction of the efferent arteriole and also may directly cause mesangial proliferation and raise GFB permeability.[4]

Metabolic Derangements

Various metabolic derangements may result in DKD. Hyperglycemia, especially in the context of oxidative stress and dyslipidemia, can directly modify proteins and contribute to GFB permeability, mesangial expansion, and glomerular inflammation. Additionally, increased glycolysis in itself has deleterious consequences, including raising susceptibility to oxidative stress, promoting cytokine-mediated mesangial expansion, and worsening hyperfiltration injury.[4,5]

Immune Dysregulation

Hyperglycemia is associated with an up-regulation of proinflammatory and profibrotic pathways that result in GFB damage, mesangial expansion, and tubulointerstitial fibrosis. Importantly, podocyte turnover (a crucial process in maintaining the GFB) also is impaired by hyperglycemia.[4–6]

Effect on the Glomerular Filtration Barrier

The mechanisms, described previously, progressively lead to GFB damage, lower GFR, and albuminuria. Albuminuria rises with GFB damage and may contribute independently to downstream tubulointerstitial fibrosis. Thus, albuminuria is both a hallmark of and a risk factor for DKD progression.[6]

NATURAL HISTORY

The risks of development and progression of DKD primarily depend on the duration of diabetes, glycemic control, and hypertension control.[7,8] For T2DM, approximately 30% of patients develop microalbuminuria within 10 years of diabetes diagnosis, and approximately 5% progress to overt nephropathy every year.[7] Nearly all patients with low GFR from DKD have preceding albuminuria, and the degree of albuminuria predicts the rate of GFR decline.[8-11] Effective hyperglycemia and hypertension management can delay the onset of microalbuminuria and slow DKD progression. For T1DM, the typical progression of DKD is summarized in **Table 1**.

All-cause mortality increases as DKD progresses, primarily from cardiovascular diseases (CVD).[7] According to the data on T2DM from the United Kingdom Prospective Diabetes Study (UKPDS), the annual rate of CVD-mortality is 0.7% for those without DKD, 2% for those with microalbuminuria, 3.5% for those with macroalbuminuria, and 12.1% for those with low GFR or kidney failure.[7] The degree of albuminuria is a predictor of poor CVD outcomes, and reduction in albuminuria has cardioprotective effects.[12]

SCREENING, MONITORING, AND DIAGNOSING DIABETIC KIDNEY DISEASE

Given the high morbidity and mortality associated with DKD, effective screening is critical. The 2019 American Diabetes Association guidelines recommend yearly assessment of GFR and albuminuria via a spot urine albumin–to–creatinine ratio (UACR) in all patients with T2DM and those with T1DM for greater than or equal to 5 years.[13] Despite this, less than or equal to 50% of patients with diabetes are tested for albuminuria.[2,13,14] Albuminuria should be screened, and, if elevated, confirmed on a separate measurement within 6 months, with microalbuminuria defined as UACR of 30 mg/g to 300 mg/g and macroalbuminuria defined as UACR greater than or equal to 300 mg/g. The presence of UACR greater than or equal to 30 mg/g or estimated GFR (eGFR) less than 60 mL/min/1.73 m^2 for at least 3 months is required for the diagnosis of DKD.[15]

NEPHROLOGY CONSULT/REFERRAL

Approximately 20% of patients with kidney failure from diabetes progress to needing dialysis without receiving care by a nephrologist.[16] Current guidelines recommend referral to nephrology when eGFR decreases below 30 mL/min/1.73 m^2, when the etiology of CKD is in question, or when there are management challenges (resistant hypertension, worsening albuminuria, rapidly declining GFR, and forth).[17] Consultation with a nephrologist should be sought prior to requesting a kidney biopsy. A longer duration of predialysis nephrology care is associated with better patient readiness for dialysis and greater 1-year survival after dialysis initiation.[18]

EVIDENCE-BASED MANAGEMENT

Optimal management of hyperglycemia, blood pressure (BP), and albuminuria is the cornerstone of evidence-based DKD management. More recently, sodium-glucose cotransporter 2 inhibitors (SGLT2Is) and glucagon-like peptide-1 (GLP-1) analogues, agents developed for blood glucose control, have emerged as important agents for DKD management, because they have been shown to slow DKD progression independent of their effect on glucose lowering.[13] The results of major clinical trials in DKD are summarized in **Table 2**. The evidence-based management approach for DKD is summarized in **Table 3** and reviewed.[2,14,19,20]

Table 1
Typical progression of diabetic kidney disease due to type 1 diabetes mellitus

	Diagnosis of Diabetes	Incipient Diabetic Kidney Disease	Overt Diabetic Kidney Disease	End-stage Kidney Disease
Time since the onset of diabetes	0–5 y	5–15 y	15–25 y	25–30 y
Kidney Function	↑ in GFR	Normal GFR	Progressive ↓ in GFR	GFR <15 mL/min
Albuminuria	Normal albuminuria, or intermittent microalbuminuria	Intermittent microalbuminuria to persistent microalbuminuria	Macroalbuminuria to nephrotic range albuminuria	Variable— ↓ albuminuria with the ↓ in the number of functional nephrons
Main kidney pathology findings	Normal kidney architecture, or glomerular hypertrophy	Mesangial expansion, glomerular basement membrane thickening, focal mesangial sclerosis	Marked glomerular basement membrane thickening, nodular glomerulosclerosis (Kimmelstiel-Wilson lesions), tubulointerstitial fibrosis

Table 2
Landmark trials in diabetic kidney disease management

Study (y)	Average Follow-up (mo)	Baseline Characteristics	Intervention	Comparator	Main Findings
Type 1 diabetes mellitus					
Collaborative Study Group (1993) N = 409	36	sCr: 1.3 mg/dL HbA$_{1c}$: 11.8% Albuminuria: 2.5 g/d	Captopril	Placebo	Captopril ↓ time to doubling of sCr by 43%
Type 2 diabetes mellitus					
IDNT (2001) N = 1715	31	sCr: 1.7 mg/dL HbA$_{1c}$: 8.1% Albuminuria: 2.9 g/d	Irbesartan	Amlodipine, Placebo	Irbesartan ↓ risk of doubling of sCr, death, or progression to kidney failure by 20% compared with placebo and 23% compared with amlodipine
RENAAL (2001) N = 1513	41	sCr: 1.9 mg/dL HbA$_{1c}$: 8.4% Albuminuria: 1.2 g/d	Losartan	Placebo	Losartan ↓ risk of doubling of sCr, death, or progression to kidney failure.
EMPAREG (2015) N = 7020	37	eGFR: 82 mL/min/1.73 m^2 HbA$_{1c}$: 8.1% 40% with micro/ macroalbuminuria	Empagliflozin	Placebo	Empagliflozin ↓ risk of incident or worsening nephropathy, progression to macroalbuminuria, doubling of sCr, or time to kidney failure
CANVAS (2017) N = 10,142	43	eGFR: 76 mL/min/1.73 m^2 HbA$_{1c}$: 8.2% UACR: 12.3 mg/g	Canagliflozin	Placebo	Canagliflozin ↓ progression of albuminuria and risk of eGFR reduction, kidney failure, or death from renal cause
CREDENCE (2019) N = 4401	31	eGFR: 56 mL/min/1.73 m^2 HbA$_{1c}$: 8.3% UACR: 923 mg/g	Canagliflozin	Placebo	Canagliflozin ↓ risk of doubling of sCr, kidney failure, or death from kidney or cardiovascular causes

(continued on next page)

Table 2
(continued)

Study (y)	Average Follow-up (mo)	Baseline Characteristics	Intervention	Comparator	Main Findings
LEADER (2016) N = 9340	46	eGFR: 80 mL/min/1.73 m^2 HbA$_{1c}$: 8.7% 37% with micro/ macroalbuminuria	Liraglutide	Placebo	Liraglutide ↓ risk of new onset persistent macroalbuminuria, doubling of sCr, kidney failure, death from kidney causes
REWIND (2019) N = 9901	65	eGFR: 77 mL/min/1.73 m^2 HbA$_{1c}$: 7.3% 35% with micro/ macroalbuminuria	Dulaglutide	Placebo	Dulaglutide ↓ risk of new macroalbuminuria, decrease in eGFR by 30%, and kidney failure

Abbreviation: N, number; sCr, serum creatinine.

Table 3
Clinical management of diabetic kidney disease

Patient Group	Suggested Interventions
Everyone with DKD	• Hyperglycemia management targeting HbA$_{1c}$ ≤7.0%, if not limited by hypoglycemia episodes • Dyslipidemia management per standard guidelines for patients with diabetes • Dietary counseling for those who are overweight or obese, including referral to intensive behavioral counseling interventions or weight management programs • Reducing salt intake to <2 g of sodium (corresponding to 5 g of sodium chloride) per day • Smoking cessation counseling and treatment, if applicable • Avoiding potentially nephrotoxic insults whenever possible • Nephrology referral if GFR is <30 mL/1.73 m² or if an alternate cause of kidney disease is suspected

DKD with hypertension	• Targeting BP of <130/80 mm Hg, adding these medications in a stepwise fashion:
	  ○ ACEI or ARB as first-line agents
	  ○ Diuretics and/or calcium channel blockers as second/third line if BP goal is not achieved with ACEI or ARB
	  ○ Spironolactone if still not at goal and GFR >30 mL/min/1.73 m², unless limited by hyperkalemia
	• Nephrology referral if BP control is not achieved with 4 agents

DKD with UACR ≥30 mg/g without hypertension	• Consideration of ACEI or ARB, if not limited by side effects, if 1 of the following is present:
	  ○ Increasing levels of albuminuria over time
	  ○ Declining GFR
	  ○ Presence of retinopathy, hyperlipidemia, or hyperuricemia
	  ○ Family history of hypertension, macrovascular disease, or DKD
	• Consideration for SGLT2I if UACR >300 mg/g and GFR ≥30 mL/min/1.73 m²

DKD with UACR ≥30 mg/g and hypertension	• Management of hypertension, as noted previously • Up-titration of ACEI/ARB dosage (maximum dosage: 80 mg of lisinopril equivalent or 200 mg of losartan equivalent) to achieve maximum albuminuria reduction as tolerated by BP and side effects • SGLT2I in addition to ACEI or ARB if UACR >300 mg/g and GFR ≥30 mL/min/1.73 m² • Spironolactone in addition to the maximum tolerated dose of ACEI or ARB if UACR remains ≥300 mg/g and if GFR >30 mL/min/1.73 m², unless limited by hyperkalemia

Glycemic Control

Achieving and maintaining euglycemia are crucial elements in avoiding the onset and progression of DKD related to both T1DM and T2DM. Several studies have demonstrated the benefit of adequate glycemic control as it pertains to the development of microvascular complications. In the landmark Diabetes Control and Complications Trial (DCCT), 1993, improved glycemic control (hemoglobin A$_{1C}$ [HbA$_{1C}$]) <6% versus around 9%) in patients with T1DM without DKD was associated with 39% reduction in the rate of microalbuminuria and 54% reduction in the rate of macroalbuminuria over 6.5 years of follow-up.[21] Although the original trial did not show any benefit for hard

CKD-related or CVD-related outcomes, the long-term follow-up of DCCT participants showed 42% lower rate of CVD over 10 years and 50% lower rate of CKD over 22-year in the intensive glucose control group.[22,23] Similarly, for T2DM, aggressive glycemic control was associated with a significantly lower rate of microvascular complications in the UKPDS trial.[24] The Action to Control Cardiovascular Risk in Diabetes trial (ACCORD), 2008; the Action in Diabetes and Vascular Disease: Preterax and Diamicron Modified Release Controlled Evaluation (ADVANCE) trial, 2008; and the Veterans Affairs Diabetes Trial (VADT), 2009, are 3 large trials in T2DM investigating glycemic control and CVD outcomes that also have secondarily examined kidney outcomes. Of these, only ADVANCE demonstrated an association between lower HbA_{1c} target (6.3% vs 7.0%) and improved kidney outcomes.[25–27]

Although this is primarily a discussion of glycemic control in the context of DKD, it is relevant to discuss the relationship between tight glycemic control and cardiovascular outcomes, given the co-occurrence of DKD and CVD. ACCORD, ADVANCE, and VADT all included patients at high cardiovascular risks and compared cardiovascular outcomes in individuals with strict versus conventional glycemic control. In ACCORD, strict control (target HbA_{1c} <6% vs HbA_{1c} 7%–7.9%) was associated with a higher risk of mortality, and subgroup analysis demonstrated elevated risk in participants with a prior history of CVD.[25] The ADVANCE and VADT trials did not demonstrate an elevated cardiovascular risk with strict HbA_{1c} targets (6.3% and 6.9%, respectively); however, there was a significantly higher risk of hypoglycemia without any appreciable cardiovascular benefit.[25–27] Overall, the results of these trials raise a concern that a very strict glycemic control may result in harm without improving macrovascular complications in T2DM.

Comorbidities, drug metabolism, and side-effect profile are some of the factors that need to be taken into consideration when selecting a glucose-lowering medication for patients with DKD. Certain sulfonylureas that are cleared by kidneys, in particular glyburide, glibenclamide, and glimepiride, should be used with caution in individuals with CKD due to the risk for severe hypoglycemia. Glipizide and gliclazide are cleared primarily by the liver and are relatively safer. Although thiazolidinediones are metabolized by the cytochrome P450 system and do not exhibit excess hypoglycemia in DKD patients, they should be used with caution in DKD due to their association with fluid retention, anemia, and osteoporosis. Kidneys are involved in one-third of exogenous insulin degradation and it is important to reduce insulin dosage and have a higher vigilance for hypoglycemia in patients with advanced DKD. Metformin, SGLT2I, and GLP-1 analogues (GLP-1As) are discussed in detail later, given their specific implications for DKD.

Although kidney disease and diabetes guidelines recommend a target HbA_{1c} of 7.0% in patients with DKD, patient comorbidities need to be taken into consideration, and the known benefit of aggressive diabetes control for kidney outcomes needs to be balanced with the risks of hypoglycemia and CVD events.[2,13,14] Thus, it is recommended that the goal HbA_{1c} be individualized for each patient.

Blood Pressure Control

BP control slows DKD progression and decreases cardiovascular mortality.[28–31] Despite the evidence that lower BP slows DKD progression, the BP goal for patients with diabetes is somewhat controversial. The Systolic Blood Pressure Intervention Trial, 2015, demonstrated that in patients with high cardiovascular risk, lower target BP (systolic BP <120 vs <140) is associated with improved cardiovascular and all-cause mortality.[32] These results, however, are not directly applicable to patients with diabetes because they were excluded from the trial. The ACCORD-Blood

Pressure study investigated the effect of strict BP control on cardiovascular outcomes specifically in patients with diabetes and high CVD risk. Results demonstrated that a lower BP target (systolic BP <120 vs <140) was associated with a lower risk for albuminuria progression and stroke without any benefit for composite fatal and nonfatal CVD events over 5 years of follow-up.[29] Serious adverse events attributable to antihypertensive treatment were more common in the low BP arm (3.3% vs 1.3%). In midst of these uncertainties, current guidelines recommend a BP goal of less than 130/80 for patients with diabetes.[33]

Renin-Angiotensin-Aldosterone System Blockade

Blockade of RAAS is a mainstay strategy in the management of DKD. The benefit of RAAS blockade in DKD is independent of BP lowering and likely is primarily from lowering of intraglomerular pressure and the resultant hyperfiltration injury and albuminuria. Because albuminuria reduction is linked with slowing DKD progression and improving CVD outcomes, controlling albuminuria is an important goal in DKD management.[30,34] Angiotensin-converting enzymes inhibitors (ACEIs), angiotensin-II receptor blockers (ARBs), mineralocorticoid antagonists, and direct renin inhibitors (DRIs) are major RAAS blockers studied in DKD.

Large trials (see **Table 2**) demonstrating the efficacy of RAAS blockade in the treatment of DKD were published as early as 1993, when captopril, independent of BP reduction, was shown to lower the risk of doubling of serum creatinine by 48% over 3 years in individuals with T1DM and high-grade albuminuria.[21] This was assessed further in subjects with T2DM and high-grade proteinuria in the Reduction of Endpoints in NIDDM with the Angiotensin II Antagonist Losartan (RENAAL) and Irbesartan Diabetic Nephropathy (IDNT) trials, which showed that, independent of BP reduction, ARB use was associated with the reduction of a composite endpoint of doubling of serum creatinine, death, and kidney failure by 16% and 20%, respecitvley, over approximately 3 years respectively.[35,36] Further analysis of RENAAL data demonstrated that those with a higher baseline albuminuria (UACR ≥3 g/g) were at a much higher risk of progressing to kidney failure.[37] Similarly, the same analysis showed that the reduction in albuminuria was proportionally related to kidney protection, with every 50% reduction in albuminuria in the first 6 months of the trial being associated with a 45% reduction in the risk for kidney failure during approximately 3-year of subsequent follow-up. These results have been replicated in post hoc analysis of other large trials.[38]

Up to a 30% rise in serum creatinine is expected shortly after ACEI/ARB initiation becaus the decrease in intraglomerular pressure also leads to decrease in creatinine clearance. ACEI/ARB, however, should not be stopped with this initial rise in serum creatinine because the long-term rate of GFR decline slows with ACEI/ARB use.[21,35,36] Even then, it is reasonable to check serum creatinine and potassium values within 2 weeks of ACEI/ARB initiation because patients with coexisting renovascular disease may exhibit higher than expected increase in serum creatinine or hyperkalemia. If greater than 30% rise in serum creatinine or hyperkalemia is noted, then it is reasonable to refer the patient to a nephrologist and stop ACEI/ARB. Likewise, the risk for hyperkalemia increases in individuals with eGFR of less than 30 mL/min/1.73 m². Although ACEI/ARB has been shown to delay the onset of kidney failure even in people with eGFR of 15 mL/min/1.73m² to 30 mL/min/1.73 m², it is prudent to refer patients with advanced CKD to a nephrologist to closely manage potential hyperkalemia and to initiate preparation for renal replacement therapy.[39]

There is some evidence that patients with diabetes may benefit from ACEI/ARB prior to the development of albuminuria. Ruggenenti and colleagues[40] investigated the effect of RAAS blockade on patients with T2DM and hypertension without microalbuminuria and found that ACEI treatment delayed the onset of microalbuminuria. In addition, preemptive use of ACEI in patients with T2DM without hypertension or microalbuminuria also has been shown to attenuate the decline in kidney function and reduce the absolute level of albuminuria.[41] Given the lack of hard outcome data, however, preemptive ACEI/ARB is not currently recommended in clinical practice guidelines.

Use of more than 1 class of RAAS blockers in combination has been studied in DKD. ACEI plus ARB therapy compared with monotherapy consistently has been shown to lower BP and proteinuria but raises the risk for significant adverse events.[19,42–49] DRIs in combination with ACEI/ARB also have been shown to modestly improve BP and proteinuria without affecting clinical CVD and kidney endpoints, resulting in higher rates of severe adverse events like hyperkalemia and hypotension.[50,51] In 1 study, combining spironolactone with ACEI was found to slow albuminuria progression compared with ACEI plus ARB combination without significantly increasing adverse effects.[19] The safety and efficacy of this combination, however, have not been assessed further in well-powered trials. In view of these data, ACEI plus ARB and DRI plus ACEI/ARB combinations should not be used in DKD; spironolactone plus ACEI/ARB can be considered in refractory cases of high-grade proteinuria as long as GFR is not less than 30 mL/min/1.73 m^2 given the risk for hyperkalemia, and DRI or spironolactone alone should be considered only if patients have significant intolerance to ACEI/ARBs.

Although post hoc analyses of trials suggest that reduction in albuminuria proportionally confers kidney protection, the specific albuminuria target is an area of uncertainty. Until a specific albuminuria target is better defined in clinical trials, it is reasonable to use ACEI/ARB to lower BP to at least less than 130/80 mm Hg and achieve maximum albuminuria reduction as tolerated by BP and side effects. In addition, there is evidence that high salt intake may reduce the antiproteinuric effect of RAAS blockade, so the importance of a low-salt diet should be emphasized to all patients with DKD.[52]

Metformin

Metformin remains the foundation of antiglycemic therapy in clinical practice guidelines, with demonstrated benefits to patients with and without CKD.[53] Historically, concern for metformin provoking lactic acidosis lead to its avoidance in patients with CKD, but, since 2010, several studies have shown that there is no increase in lactic acidosis in patients with mild to moderate kidney impairment, and metformin potentially may confer a mortality benefit.[54,55] These recent studies ultimately led the Food Drug Administration to update metformin labeling in 2016. The current labeling supports metformin initiation in patients with an eGFR of greater than 45 mL/min/1.73 m^2 and continuation (but not initiation) in patients whose eGFR fall between 30 mL/min/1.73 m^2 and 45 mL/min/1.73 m^2 if the risk outweighs the benefits (possibly with a dose reduction) and considers an eGFR of less than 30 mL/min/1.73 m^2 a contraindication to metformin use.[56] Metformin does not have a well-demonstrated impact on the progression of DKD beyond its reduction in hyperglycemia, but, given a possible mortality benefit, it should be used when feasible in patients with T2DM.

Sodium-glucose Cotransporter 2 Inhibitors

SGLT2Is in the proximal tubule have been a known therapeutic target for glucose-lowering since 2013. More recently, SGLT2Is, also known as gliflozins, have been shown to have cardioprotective and kidney-protective effects independent of glucose lowering (see **Table 2**).

The Empagliflozin, Cardiovascular Outcomes, and Mortality in Type 2 Diabetes (EMPAREG) was the first large trial to show that empagliflozin not only reduced CVD outcomes, the trial's primary endpoint, but also slowed DKD progression.[57,58] Follow-up studies, including the Canagliflozin Cardiovascular Assessment Study (CANVAS) and the Dapagliflozin Effect on Cardiovascular Events–Thrombolysis in Myocardial Infarction 58 (DECLARE-TIMI 58) trial, also supported the idea that this class of medication could slow DKD progression.[59–61] These early trials, however, were not specifically powered to detect kidney outcomes.

The Canagliflozin and Renal Outcomes in Type 2 Diabetes and Nephropathy (CREDENCE) was the first trial specifically powered to assess kidney outcomes in participants with T2DM who already were on a maximal tolerated dose of ACEI/ARB.[62] In this large trial involving greater than 4000 high-risk participants followed over 2.5 years, the risk for composite outcome of doubling of serum creatinine level, kidney failure, or death from kidney or cardiovascular causes was 30% lower in the canagliflozin group compared with placebo, resulting in the number needed to treat of 22 to prevent 1 major outcome. Rates of severe adverse events were similar in 2 groups, although the rates of diabetic ketoacidosis, although low, were higher in the canagliflozin arm (2.2 vs 0.2, respectively, per 1000 patient-years).

The renoprotective mechanism for SGLT2Is is thought to be multifactorial.[63] SGLT2Is increases sodium and glucose delivery to the distal tubule, resulting in tubuloglomerular feedback that leads to afferent arteriolar vasoconstriction and reduction in intraglomerular pressure (similar to RAAS blockers). SGLT2Is also may have anti-inflammatory mechanisms and improve intrarenal oxygenation.

SGLT2Is consistently have shown remarkable cardiorenal benefits in multiple large trials, and, since the publication of the CREDENCE study, the use of SGLT2Is is becoming the standard of care adjunct to RAAS blockers for patients with T2DM and mild to moderate CKD (estimated GFR >30 mL/min/1.73 m^2) and UACR of greater than 300 mg/g.[13] Patients initiated on these agents should be counseled to be vigilant about urinary infections, in particular mycotic infections, given the inevitable glycosuria that occurs with these agents. In addition, patients also should be educated on symptoms of diabetic ketoacidosis, and it is reasonable to hold the drug if patients were to develop any systemic illness or conditions that would limit oral intake or result in significant volume loss. Further studies are under way to assess the effect of SGLT2Is in patients with T1DM.

Glucagon-like Peptide-1 Receptor Analogues

GLP-1 receptor analogues are relatively new medications that also have shown promise in slowing DKD progression, independent of their glucose-lowering effect. Trials, such as the Liraglutide Effect and Action in Diabetes: Evaluation of Cardiovascular Outcome Results (LEADER), Researching Cardiovascular Events with a Weekly Incretin in Diabetes (REWIND), and Assessment of Weekly Administration of Dulaglutide in Diabetes 7 trials have shown reduction in CVD outcomes as well as greater than 25% decreased risk of new-onset persistent macroalbuminuria over 3.8 years in T2DM participants with high CVD risk.[64–68] The mechanism for renoprotection with these agents is unclear and may be related to reduction in both oxidative stress and inflammation.[69] Although guidelines suggest GLP-1A as an add-on to metformin in patients with atherosclerotic CVD, GLP-1A also can be considered as a possible adjunct to metformin and SGL2I in patients with DKD from T2DM.[53]

SUMMARY

The morbidity and mortality associated with diabetes are both intimately linked to the evolution of DKD. Primary care physicians treat a large number of patients with diabetes and must remain vigilant in their efforts to screen for the development of DKD and make it a priority to manage DKD with an evidence-based approach targeting effective BP and glycemic control, RAAS blockade, and, when appropriate, sodium-glucose cotransporter 2 inhibition or GLP-1 receptor agonism.

DISCLOSURE

The authors have nothing to disclose.

REFERENCES

1. United States Renal Data System. 2018 USRDS annual data report: CKD in the general population. Bethesda, MD: United States Renal Data System; 2018. p. 1–28.
2. National Kidney Foundation. KDOQI clinical practice guideline for diabetes and CKD: 2012 update. Am J Kidney Dis 2012;60(5):850–86.
3. United States Renal Data System. Bethesda (MD). USRDS 2018 annual data report - Chapter 5: Mortality. United States Ren Data Syst 2018 USRDS Annu data Rep Epidemiol kidney Dis United States Natl Institutes Heal Natl Inst Diabetes Dig Kidney Dis, vol. 2, 2018. p. 411–26. Available at: https://www.usrds.org/2018/download/v2_c05_Mortality_18_usrds.pdf.
4. Toth-Manikowski S, Atta MG. Diabetic kidney disease: Pathophysiology and therapeutic targets. J Diabetes Res 2015;2015. https://doi.org/10.1155/2015/697010.
5. Giacco F, Brownlee M. Oxidative stress and diabetic complications. Circ Res 2011;107(9):1058–70.
6. Vallon V, Komers R. Pathophysiology of the Diabetic Kidney. Compr Physiol 2011; 1(3):1175–232.
7. Adler AI, Stevens RJ, Manley SE, et al. Development and progression of nephropathy in type 2 diabetes: The United Kingdom Prospective Diabetes Study (UKPDS 64). Kidney Int 2003;63(1):225–32.
8. Gæde P, Tarnow L, Vedel P, et al. Remission to normoalbuminuria during multifactorial treatment preserves kidney function in patients with type 2 diabetes and microalbuminuria. Nephrol Dial Transplant 2004;19(11):2784–8.
9. Costacou T, Ellis D, Fried L, et al. Sequence of Progression of Albuminuria and Decreased GFR in Persons With Type 1 Diabetes: A Cohort Study. Am J Kidney Dis 2007;50(5):721–32.
10. Kunzelman CL, Knowler WC, Pettitt DJ, et al. Incidence of proteinuria in type 2 diabetes mellitus in the Pima Indians. Kidney Int 1989;35(2):681–7.
11. Nelson RG, Bennett PH, Beck GJ, et al. Development and Progression of Renal Disease in Pima Indians with Non-Insulin-Dependent Diabetes Mellitus. N Engl J Med 1996;335(22):1636–42.
12. de Zeeuw D, Remuzzi G, Parving H-H, et al. Albuminuria, a Therapeutic Target for Cardiovascular Protection in Type 2 Diabetic Patients With Nephropathy. Circulation 2004;110(8):921–7.
13. American Diabetes Association. 11. Microvascular complications and foot care: Standards of Medical Care in Diabetes - 2019. Diabetes Care 2019;42:S124–38.
14. Molitch ME, Adler AI, Flyvbjerg A, et al. Diabetic kidney disease: a clinical update from Kidney Disease: Improving Global Outcomes. Kidney Int 2015;87(1):20–30.

15. Kidney Disease Improving Global Outcomes. KDIGO 2012 Clinical Practice Guideline for the Evaluation and Management of Chronic Kidney Disease. Kidney Int 2013;3(1):1–150.

16. United States Renal Data System. USRDS Annual Data Report: Incidence, prevalence, patient characteristics, and treatment modalities. Am J Kidney Dis 2018; 59(1 SUPPL. 1). https://doi.org/10.1053/j.ajkd.2011.10.027.

17. American Diabetes Association. Standards of Medical Care in Diabetes—2019 Abridged for Primary Care Providers. Clin Diabetes 2019;37(1):11–34.

18. Gillespie BW, Morgenstern H, Hedgeman E, et al. Nephrology care prior to end-stage renal disease and outcomes among new ESRD patients in the USA. Clin Kidney J 2015;8(6):772–80.

19. Mehdi UF, Adams-Huet B, Raskin P, et al. Addition of angiotensin receptor blockade or mineralocorticoid antagonism to maximal angiotensin-converting enzyme inhibition in diabetic nephropathy. J Am Soc Nephrol 2009;20(12): 2641–50.

20. U.S. Preventative Services Task Force. Healthful Diet and Physical Activity for Cardiovascular Disease Prevention in Adults With Cardiovascular Risk Factors: Behavioral Counseling. 2016. Available at: https://www.uspreventiveservicestaskforce. org/Page/Document/RecommendationStatementFinal/healthy-diet-and-physical-activity-counseling-adults-with-high-risk-of-cvd#consider. Accessed December 1, 2019.

21. The DCCT Research Group. The Effect of Intensive Treatment of Diabetes on the Development and Progression of Long-Term Complications in Insulin-Dependent Diabetes Mellitus. N Engl J Med 1993;329(14):977–86.

22. Nathan DM, Cleary PA, Backlund J-YC, et al. Intensive diabetes treatment and cardiovascular disease in patients with type 1 diabetes. N Engl J Med 2005; 353(25):2643–53.

23. DCCT/EDIC Research Group, de Boer IH, Sun W, Cleary PA, et al. Intensive diabetes therapy and glomerular filtration rate in type 1 diabetes. N Engl J Med 2011;365(25):2366–76.

24. The UKPDS Group. Intensive blood-glucose control with sulphonylureas or insulin compared with conventional treatment and risk of complications in patients with type 2 diabetes (UKPDS 33). Lancet 1998;352(9131):837–53.

25. The ACCORD Study Group. Effects of Intensive Glucose Lowering in Type 2 Diabetes. N Engl J Med 2008;358(24):2545–59.

26. Advance Collaborative Group. Intensive Blood Glucose Control and Vascular Outcomes in Patients with Type 2 Diabetes. N Engl J Med 2008;358(24):2560–72.

27. Duckworth W, Abraira C, Moritz T, et al. Glucose control and vascular complications in veterans with type 2 diabetes. N Engl J Med 2009;360(2):129–39.

28. Mogensen CE. Long-term antihypertensive treatment inhibiting progression of diabetic nephropathy. Br Med J 1982;285(6343):685–8.

29. The ACCORD Study Group. Effects of Intensive Blood-Pressure Control in Type 2 Diabetes Mellitus. N Engl J Med 2010;362(17):1575–85.

30. De Galan BE, Perkovic V, Ninomiya T, et al. Lowering blood pressure reduces renal events in type 2 diabetes. J Am Soc Nephrol 2009;20(4):883–92.

31. Chobanian AV, Bakris GL, Black HR, et al. Seventh report of the Joint National Committee on Prevention, Detection, Evaluation, and Treatment of High Blood Pressure. Hypertension 2003;42(6):1206–52.

32. Wright JT, Williamson JD, Whelton PK, et al. A randomized trial of intensive versus standard blood-pressure control. N Engl J Med 2015;373(22):2103–16.

33. Albert MA, Hahn EJ, Himmelfarb CD, et al. 2019 ACC/AHA Guideline on the Primary Prevention of Cardiovascular Disease: A Report of the American College of Cardiology/American Heart Association Task Force on Clinical Practice Guidelines. Circulation 2019;140. https://doi.org/10.1161/CIR.0000000000000678.

34. Schmieder RE, Mann JFE, Schumacher H, et al. Changes in Albuminuria Predict Mortality and Morbidity in Patients with Vascular Disease. J Am Soc Nephrol 2011;22(7):1353–64.

35. Lewis EJ, Hunsicker LG, Clarke WR, et al. Renoprotective Effect of the Angiotensin-Receptor Antagonist Irbesartan in Patients with Nephropathy Due to Type 2 Diabetes. N Engl J Med 2001;345(12):851–60.

36. Brenner BM, Cooper ME, de Zeeuw D, et al. Effects of losartan on renal and cardiovascular outcomes in patients with type 2 diabetes and nephropathy. N Engl J Med 2001;345(12):861–9.

37. De Zeeuw D, Remuzzi G, Parving HH, et al. Proteinuria, a target for renoprotection in patients with type 2 diabetic nephropathy: Lessons from RENAAL. Kidney Int 2004;65(6):2309–20.

38. Lambers Heerspink HJ, Gansevoort RT. Albuminuria Is an Appropriate Therapeutic Target in Patients with CKD: The Pro View. Clin J Am Soc Nephrol 2015;10(6):1079–88.

39. Hou FF, Zhang X, Zhang GH, et al. Efficacy and safety of benazepril for advanced chronic renal insufficiency. N Engl J Med 2006;354(2):131–40.

40. Ruggenenti P, Fassi A, Ilieva AP, et al. Preventing Microalbuminuria in Type 2 Diabetes. N Engl J Med 2004;351(19):1941–51.

41. Ravid M, Brosh D, Levi Z, et al. Use of enalapril to attenuate decline in renal function in normotensive, normoalbuminuric patients with type 2 diabetes mellitus: A randomized, controlled trial. Ann Intern Med 1998;128(12 PART 1):982–8.

42. Rutkowski B, Tylicki L. Nephroprotective action of Renin-Angiotensin-Aldosterone system blockade in chronic kidney disease patients: The landscape after ALTITUDE and VA NEPHRON-D trails. J Ren Nutr 2015;25(2):194–200.

43. The ONTARGET Investigators. Telmisartan, Ramipril, or Both in Patients at High Risk for Vascular Events. N Engl J Med 2008;358(15):1547–59.

44. Mann JF, Schmieder RE, McQueen M, et al. Renal outcomes with telmisartan, ramipril, or both, in people at high vascular risk (the ONTARGET study): a multi-centre, randomised, double-blind, controlled trial. Lancet 2008;372(9638):547–53.

45. Fried LF, Emanuele N, Zhang JH, et al. Combined Angiotensin Inhibition for the Treatment of Diabetic Nephropathy. N Engl J Med 2013;369(20):1892–903.

46. Jacobsen P, Andersen S, Jensen BR, et al. Additive effect of ACE inhibition and Angiotensin II receptor blockade in type I diabetic patients with diabetic nephropathy. J Am Soc Nephrol 2003;14(4):992–9.

47. Jacobsen P, Andersen S, Rossing K, et al. Dual blockade of the renin-angiotensin system versus maximal recommended dose of ACE inhibition in diabetic nephropathy. Kidney Int 2003;63(5):1874–80.

48. Rossing K, Jacobsen P, Pietraszek L, et al. Renoprotective effects of adding angiotensin II receptor blocker to maximal recommended doses of ACE inhibitor in diabetic nephropathy: A randomized double-blind crossover trial. Diabetes Care 2003;26(8):2268–74.

49. Rossing K, Christensen PK, Jensen BR, et al. Dual Blockade of the Renin-Angiotensin System in Diabetic Nephropathy: A randomized double-blind cross-over study. Diabetes Care 2002;25(1):95–100.

50. Parving H-H, Brenner BM, McMurray JJV, et al. Cardiorenal End Points in a Trial of Aliskiren for Type 2 Diabetes. N Engl J Med 2012;367(23):2204–13.

51. Parving H-H, Persson F, Lewis JB, et al. Aliskiren Combined with Losartan in Type 2 Diabetes and Nephropathy. N Engl J Med 2008;358(23):2433–46.
52. Heeg JE, de Jong PE, van der Hem GK, et al. Efficacy and variability of the anti-proteinuric effect of ACE inhibition by lisinopril. Kidney Int 1989;36(2):272–9.
53. American Diabetes Association. 9. Pharmacologic Approaches to Glycemic Treatment: Standards of Medical Care in Diabetes—2019. Diabetes Care 2019; 42(Supplement 1):S90–102.
54. Crowley MJ, Diamantidis CJ, McDuffie JR, et al. Clinical Outcomes of Metformin Use in Populations With Chronic Kidney Disease, Congestive Heart Failure, or Chronic Liver Disease: A Systematic Review. Ann Intern Med 2017;166(3):191–200.
55. Lu WR, Defilippi J, Braun A. Unleash metformin: reconsideration of the contraindication in patients with renal impairment. Ann Pharmacother 2013;47(11):1488–97.
56. U.S. Food and Drug Administration. FDA Drug Safety Communication: FDA revises warnings regarding use of the diabetes medicine metformin in certain patients with reduced kidney function. 2017. Available at: https://www.fda.gov/drugs/drug-safety-and-availability/fda-drug-safety-communication-fda-revises-warnings-regarding-use-diabetes-medicine-metformin-certain. Accessed December 1, 2019.
57. Zinman B, Wanner C, Lachin JM, et al. Empagliflozin, Cardiovascular Outcomes, and Mortality in Type 2 Diabetes. N Engl J Med 2015;373(22):2117–28.
58. Wanner C, Inzucchi SE, Lachin JM, et al. Empagliflozin and Progression of Kidney Disease in Type 2 Diabetes. N Engl J Med 2016;375(4):323–34.
59. Wiviott SD, Raz I, Bonaca MP, et al. Dapagliflozin and cardiovascular outcomes in type 2 diabetes. N Engl J Med 2019;380(4):347–57.
60. Neal B, Perkovic V, Mahaffey KW, et al. CANVAS Programme Collaborative Group. Canagliflozin and Cardiovascular and Renal Events in Type 2 Diabetes. N Engl J Med 2017;130(2):149–53.
61. Bakris GL. Major Advancements in Slowing Diabetic Kidney Disease Progression: Focus on SGLT2 Inhibitors. Am J Kidney Dis 2019;74(5):573–5.
62. Perkovic V, Jardine MJ, Neal B, et al. Canagliflozin and renal outcomes in type 2 diabetes and nephropathy. N Engl J Med 2019;380(24):2295–306.
63. Ingelfinger JR, Rosen CJ. Clinical Credence - SGLT2 Inhibitors, Diabetes, and Chronic Kidney Disease. N Engl J Med 2019;380(24):2371–3.
64. Tuttle KR, Lakshmanan MC, Rayner B, et al. Dulaglutide versus insulin glargine in patients with type 2 diabetes and moderate-to-severe chronic kidney disease (AWARD-7): a multicentre, open-label, randomised trial. Lancet Diabetes Endocrinol 2018;6(8):605–17.
65. Gerstein HC, Colhoun HM, Dagenais GR, et al. Dulaglutide and cardiovascular outcomes in type 2 diabetes (REWIND): a double-blind, randomised placebo-controlled trial. Lancet 2019;394(10193):121–30.
66. Gerstein HC, Colhoun HM, Dagenais GR, et al. Dulaglutide and renal outcomes in type 2 diabetes: an exploratory analysis of the REWIND randomised, placebo-controlled trial. Lancet 2019;394(10193):131–8.
67. Mann JFE, Ørsted DD, Brown-Frandsen K, et al. Liraglutide and Renal Outcomes in Type 2 Diabetes. N Engl J Med 2017;377(9):839–48.
68. Marso SP, Daniels GH, Brown-Frandsen K, et al. Liraglutide and Cardiovascular Outcomes in Type 2 Diabetes. N Engl J Med 2016;375(4):311–22.
69. Fujita H, Morii T, Fujishima H, et al. The protective roles of GLP-1R signaling in diabetic nephropathy: possible mechanism and therapeutic potential. Kidney Int 2014;85(3):579–89.

Nephrolithiasis

Kelley Bishop, MD*, Tobe Momah, MD, Janet Ricks, DO

KEYWORDS

- Nephrolithiasis • Urolithiasis • Hematuria • Kidney stone • Calcium oxalate

KEY POINTS

- Kidney stones, which may asymptomatic or cause significant pain and other systemic symptoms, present both acutely and chronically and in various ureteral locations.
- Etiology of stones can arise from genetic or environmental factors, with diagnosis based on symptoms, laboratory work, and imaging.
- Treatment of nephrolithiasis is multifactorial and should address nutrition and hydration status as well as medical or surgical management.
- Complications should be identified and managed quickly to minimize permanent kidney damage.
- Referral to specialist care (nephrology or urology) should be considered when conservative measures have failed.

INTRODUCTION

Nephrolithiasis, otherwise referred to as kidney stones, is the most common chronic kidney condition, after hypertension.[1] The term originates from 2 Greek words: *nephros* (kidney) and *lithos* (stone)[2] and the condition is considered part of urolithiasis (stones in urine), alongside ureterolithiasis (stones in ureter) and cystolithiasis (stones in the urinary bladder).

The first case documented in the literature was reported between 3200 BCE and 1200 BCE.[3] Stones typically develop in the kidney and pass through the urine. Although some are asymptomatic, others may grow to the point that they obstruct the ureters, causing significant discomfort. Many people who have developed a kidney stone have another within a decade.[4]

INCIDENCE/PREVALENCE

The prevalence data from National Health and Nutrition Examination Survey has shown an increase in renal stones over the past few years. The most recent prevalence

---

Department of Family Medicine, University of Mississippi Medical Center, 2500 North State Street, Jackson, MS 39216, USA
* Corresponding author.
E-mail address: kbishop2@umc.edu

Prim Care Clin Office Pract 47 (2020) 661–671
https://doi.org/10.1016/j.pop.2020.08.005
0095-4543/20/© 2020 Elsevier Inc. All rights reserved.

for 2007 to 2010 has been 8.8% nationally. There has been a similar increase internationally as well. The gender difference previously seen between men and women also is decreasing; the prevalence was 10.6% for men and 7.1% for women. According to these data, renal stones affect approximately 1 in 11 people in the United States.[5] The question arises of what is causing the increase: environmental changes or improved detection of asymptomatic stones due to improved or increased use of imaging studies.

Environmental factors, such as climate and occupation, may play a part in the development of renal stones. Heat exposure and dehydration may increase the risk, primarily in men. Evaluation of insurance claims data has found that stone-related claims peaked in the hotter summer months of July to September.

Another risk that is not as well defined is the association of obesity and metabolic syndrome and renal stones. Analysis of insurance claims data found that obesity and weight gain were independent risks independent of diet. The risk increases with increasing body mass index up to 30 kg/m^2, at which time it stabilizes. The pathophysiology of this increased risk is not completely understood.[6,7]

PATHOGENESIS/PATHOPHYSIOLOGY

Renal stones develop when urine becomes supersaturated with stone-forming salts, most commonly calcium oxalate (60% of all stones), although other crystals may precipitate. If urine becomes supersaturated and no inhibition is present, then the crystals begin to form on existing surfaces of epithelial cells, cell debris, or other crystals. Several molecules assist with inhibition, such as magnesium and citrate. Nephrocalcin inhibits calcium oxalate. Tamm-Horsfall mucoprotein inhibits aggregation; uropontin inhibits crystal growth. Bikunin inhibits crystal nucleation and aggregation. There are no known specific inhibitors of uric acid crystal formation.

Calcium Stones

Hypercalciuria is the most common abnormality leading to calcium-containing stones. Hypercalciuria may occur in up to 65% of patients with stones. Abnormalities in calcium metabolism by the kidney can be divided into 3 categories: absorptive hypercalciuria (increased absorption in the intestine), renal hypercalciuria (primary renal lead of calcium), and resorptive hypercalciuria (increased bone demineralization).

Several processes may lead to increased absorption of calcium in the intestine. Increased oral calcium load suppresses parathyroid hormone and increases renal filtration of calcium with the serum calcium being normal. There also are vitamin D–dependent processes—increased vitamin D production or intake and increased sensitivity to vitamin D. Renal phosphate wasting also increases the vitamin D level.

Renal hypercalciuria is caused by impaired renal tubular reabsorption of calcium, which causes elevated urinary calcium levels and secondary hyperparathyroidism. There are several genetic mutations and abnormalities that may lead to the calcium leak: Dent disease (X-linked recessive nephrolithiasis), familial hypomagnesemia with hypercalciuria and nephrocalcinosis (mutations in claudin-16 and claudin-19), Bartter syndrome (autosomal recessive involving the loop of Henle), and autosomal dominant form of hypocalcemia (mutations in the gene encoding CaSR). Resorptive hypercalciuria is infrequent and associated commonly with primary hyperparathyroidism. Other, more rare causes of resorptive hypercalciuria are sarcoidosis, thyrotoxicosis, hypercalcemia of malignancy, and vitamin D toxicity.

Uric Acid Stones

Uric acid stones comprise 8% to 10% of all renal stones. The main determinants of uric acid stone formation are low urine pH, low urine volume, and hyperuricosuria. The most important of these is low pH. Congenital disorders involving renal tubular urate transport or uric acid metabolism lead to hyperuricosuria. Acquired causes are chronic diarrhea, volume depletion, myeloproliferative disorders, and uricosuric drugs. Uric acid stones also may develop with diets high in animal protein.

Struvite Stones

Struvite stones may be generated by urea-splitting bacteria, mycobacteria, or yeast creating urease. Urease normally is not present in human urine. The chemical cascade starts with urea (normally found in urine) and splits to urease, ultimately ending in struvite (magnesium ammonium phosphate), which can then form stones. Calcium also may adhere to struvite creating a mixed stone. The most common organisms that cause this type of stone are Proteus, Klebsiella, Pseudomonas, and Staphylococcus. Because these stones occur most commonly in people prone to frequent urinary tract infections (UTIs), women are affected more commonly than men, with a ratio of 2:1. Other comorbid states that may increase the risk are spinal cord injury, urinary tract malformation, diabetes, and urinary stasis.

Other

Other stones are rare but may include cysteine; infection stones consisting primarily of magnesium ammonium phosphate hexahydrate, xanthine, dihydroxyadenine, or ammonium acid urate; and protein matrix stones. Certain medications can precipitate in the urine and form stones; these are listed in **Table 1**. These stones generally form as crystals after taking excessive amounts of the drug.[6]

Table 1
Lithogenic drugs

Drug	Stone Formation
Atazanavir/ indinavir	Supersaturation
Acyclovir	Supersaturation
Sulfa drugs	Supersaturation
Methotrexate	Supersaturation
Triamterene	Supersaturation
Quinolones	Supersaturation
Ephedrine	Supersaturation
Magnesium trisilicate	Supersaturation
Loop diuretics	Calcium
Acetazolamide	Calcium
Zonisamide	Calcium

CLINICAL PRESENTATION

More than 40% of patients with kidney stones are asymptomatic.[5] Among the symptomatic patients, the most common presenting complaint is sudden-onset abdominal pain, cramping in nature, and associated with moderate to severe colic, also known as renal colic.[8] This pain is localized mostly to the flank or anterior upper abdomen[9] and usually occurs when the stone enters or obstructs the ureter. As the stone descends, however, it may present as pain in the ipsilateral testicle or labia.

Additional accompanying symptoms include urinary urgency, sweating, hematuria, and nausea and vomiting. Approximately 50% of nephrolithiasis patients who are symptomatic present with nausea and vomiting,[10] secondary to the shared splanchnic innervation of the renal capsule and intestines.[11] The abdominal pain, however, stops abruptly when the stone passes into the bladder, and it is not aggravated or alleviated by a change of position.

Hematuria is present in more than 90% of nephrolithiasis patients,[12] but its absence does not rule out nephrolithiasis. Individuals whose kidney stones are at the ureterovesical junction present with increased frequency of urination and dysuria[9] that could be mistaken for a UTI.

In order to differentiate nephrolithiasis from UTI, however, the patient must be evaluated for fever, chills, and cloudy foul-smelling urine. In patients with staghorn calculi, where large renal stones are impacted in the pelvis of the kidney, UTIs and obstructive symptoms that lead to permanent kidney damage and hydronephrosis could be the presenting signs and symptoms.[13]

Elderly patients with nephrolithiasis are more likely to have a subclinical presentation. They present with atypical or no pain, fever, gastrointestinal symptoms, pyuria, or UTI.[14] They also tend to have larger stone diameters and increased need for surgical intervention as they grow older. In children, on the other hand, nephrolithiasis symptoms are consistent with an adult's clinical presentation but may consist more of hematuria, generalized abdominal pain, or UTI.[1]

LABORATORY WORK-UP

Laboratory tests include urinalysis, complete blood cell count (CBC), and serum chemistry to evaluate creatinine clearance.[8] A woman of childbearing age should undergo a pregnancy test, and a CBC with differential level is indicated especially for patients with systemic signs of infection or an alternate abdominal etiology to nephrolithiasis. The most common urinalysis finding in nephrolithiasis patients is hematuria (more than 90%).[12] Other urinalysis findings seen in these patients include pyuria, leukocyte esterase, nitrites, or greater than 50 white blood cells per high-power field (if concomitant with UTI)[8] (**Box 1**).

IMAGING WORK-UP

Further radiologic testing may be necessary for establishing a diagnosis of kidney stones after initial clinical and laboratory assessment. The current gold standard for diagnosing the majority of kidney stones is the low-dose CT, with 95% sensitivity and 98% specificity. Another radiologic study that may be required in certain circumstances is the renal ultrasound, which is the usual choice in pregnant patients and in children. A drawback to renal ultrasound is that distal ureteric calculi that are less than 5 mm generally are not visible on ultrasound and the reliability is operator-dependent.[15] The intravenous pyelogram, which was the gold standard prior to the CT, in

> **Box 1**
> **Laboratory work-up**
>
> Microscopic urinalysis
> - Red blood cells, bacteria, leukocytes, urinary casts, crystals
> - Urine culture and sensitivity
>
> CBC
> - Neutrophilia (can be suggestive of struvite stones)
>
> Renal function panel/chemistry
> - Hypercalcemia
>
> Strain urine
> - Stone analysis
>
> 24-Hour urine stone risk profile
> - Determine dietary guidance/medicinal prevention

general lacks specificity and sensitivity but may be required in diagnosing radiolucent stones, such as those caused by protease inhibitors, such as indinavir.[16,17]

WORK-UP FOR RECURRENT STONES

The work-up should be considered based on a patient's risk factors and history. Taking a detailed personal and familial history can guide how extensive the initial work-up should be. Unless a patient has family or personal history of stones, a history of repetitive UTIs, a history of nephrocalcinosis, or a history of gastroenterologic disease, such as Crohn or ulcerative colitis, the diagnostic work-up assessment should consist of a urinalysis with microscopic, blood work including electrolytes and kidney function tests, serum calcium and phosphorus levels, and uric acid levels.[18]

While taking the history, a detailed dietary intake should be done as well as a complete medication intake history, focusing particularly on medications that can contribute to kidney stones[18] (see **Table 1**). Within the dietary history, a quantification of fluid intake should be documented. Other contributing diseases and conditions should be screened for in the history, such as hyperparathyroidism, renal tubular acidosis, and prior urologic surgeries.[16]

If available, collection of the stone by straining the urine can be helpful in directing prevention therapy and further diagnostic studies.[18] For patients found to have a uric acid or cystine stone, for those where a stone is unobtainable, and for patients with multiple calcium stones, studies including a 24-hour urine stone risk profile should be considered to help determine direction in dietary guidance or possible medicinal prevention[18,19] (see **Box 1**).

MANAGEMENT PRIOR TO REFERRAL

Management of acute renal calculi is determined by the presence of infection or obstruction. Larger stones, greater than 8 mm, rarely pass spontaneously and usually require urology referral. The American Urological Association recommends ureteroscopy and extracorporeal short-wave lithotripsy as first-line treatment of ureteral-placed stones and percutaneous nephrostomy if a stent is not possible.[20] Obstruction is less likely in stones less than 3 mm. Most of these calculi resolve with hydration as well as pain control.[16] Hydration should be attempted with the aim of maintaining a urine output of greater than 2 L per day.[15]

In the era of opioid crisis, effort should be made to attempt pain control without use of scheduled drugs.[21] Furthermore, nonsteroidal anti-inflammatory drugs (NSAIDs) have been shown to be equivalent or superior to opioids and/or morphine. In a 2018 systematic review and meta-analysis published by Panthan and colleagues,[22] NSAIDs were shown to be equivalent to opioids or acetaminophen for the relief of acute renal colic at 30 minutes with less vomiting and fewer requirements for rescue analgesia. Of the NSAIDs available, diclofenac was shown to be superior in a 2017 review by Garcia-Perdomo and colleagues[23] and was superior to morphine for pain reduction.

Lifestyle Modifications for Prevention of Stone Recurrence

Management of patients with history of multiple kidney stones should be centered on prevention. In this realm, management through diet is one of the most cost-effective measures. Diets high in animal protein have been shown to increase acid load, thereby reducing the urine pH, which contributes to enhancing urinary calcium excretion. Avoidance of animal protein in a diet low in meat, fish, and poultry can help achieve an alkaline urine. In addition, a diet of increased intake of fruits and vegetables high in potassium has been shown beneficial.[24,25] Alkaline urine is preferable to prevent calcium, cystine, and uric acid stones.[25] Studies have shown that reducing soft drinks or colas acidified with phosphoric acid, as well as a diet high in calcium and low in protein and sodium, reduced stone recurrence.[20] Patients with calcium oxalate stones have been counseled in times past to limit oxalate dietary intake. This has shown to be ineffective unless the patient has hyperoxaluria. Furthermore, adequate calcium dietary intake (1000–1200 mg daily) could reduce the consequences of dietary oxalate.[26] For prevention of uric acid stones in particular, limiting purine-containing foods is recommended[15] (**Box 2**).

As in acute management, hydration to maintain an adequate urine output of greater than 2 L a day is a good step in prevention.[25] In that realm, recommendation of drinking 1 beer or so a day has had mixed results in that it has been shown to be somewhat helpful in the prevention of calcium stones but may be counterproductive in prevention of urate stones.[15] The importance of the type of hydration also has been seen in several large studies in that increased stone formation was seen with increased sugar-sweetened soda, postulated to be secondary to high fructose content. Artificial sweeteners did not convey the same risk, and increased intake of coffee, tea, red and white wine, beer, and orange juice had a protective effect[24] (see **Box 2**).

Iatrogenic Consideration for Prevention of Stone Recurrence

Consideration toward iatrogenic causes must be made in the prevention of stones. Some medications that are known to be lithogenic, prone to forming crystals in the urine, are atazanavir, indinavir, acyclovir, sulfadiazine, methotrexate, triamterene,

---

Box 2
Lifestyle modification for prevention of kidney stones

- Hydration to attain urine output greater than 2 L daily
- High-calcium, high-potassium, low-protein, low-sodium diet
- Limit soft drinks acidified with phosphoric acid
- Limit purine-containing food (prevention of uric acid stones
- Limit high-fructose corn syrup intake

quinolones, sulfa medications, guaifenesin/ephedrine, and magnesium trisilicate. In addition, loop diuretics, acetazolamide, topiramate, and zonisamide all have been seen to increase incidence of calcium stones (see **Table 1**). An effort to change from these medications in patients who have been diagnosed with a stone probably formed from drug deposition should be attempted. Also, limiting ammonium acid–based laxatives is prudent in uric acid stone formers because ammonium acid urate calculi can be seen with urine supersaturation with ammonia and uric acid.[15,27]

Pharmacologic Therapy for Prevention of Stone Recurrence

Pharmacologic therapy for prevention of calcium, uric acid, and cystine stones should be considered if hydration and dietary management have been ineffective. For those types of stones, affecting an alkaline urine is recommended. This can be achieved with supplementation of potassium citrate at doses of 20 mEq to 80 mEq divided 3 times to 4 times daily with a target urinary pH of not below 6.5. Special consideration should be given to avoiding increasing the pH too far to prevent calcium phosphate supersaturation, thereby contributing to stone formation.[15]

For calcium stones, addition of thiazides and/or allopurinol has been shown protective.[20] Thiazides help in resorption of calcium at the renal tubule, especially in combination with a low-salt diet. Doses used were at least 50 mg daily.[24] Reduction of dietary sodium can decrease renal tubular calcium reabsorption, encouraging urinary excretion of calcium.[25] Studies have shown that people following the Dietary Approaches to Stop Hypertension (DASH) diet with the highest DASH scores had a 40% to 50% reduced stone formation.[24]

For uric acid stone prevention, lowering serum uric acid by addition of allopurinol is recommended if diet is not sufficient.[15] Also, uricosuric medications, such as probenecid, should be avoided, because they contribute to urinary excretion of uric acid.[25] Furthermore, hyperuricosuria has been shown to increase formation of calcium oxalate crystals in vitro, leading to the supposition that it may increase incidence of calculi in calcium oxalate stone formers. Recommended dosing for prevention is 100 mg to 300 mg daily.[15,24]

If dietary management proves insufficient in preventing cystine stones, pharmacologic therapy with medications, such as D-penicillamine and tiopronin, which bind cystine, may be considered. Although robust studies are not available, decrease of calculi formation up to 75% has been seen in a few uncontrolled and observational trials. Dosages used were 1 g/d to 2 g/d of penicillamine or 800 mg/d to 1200 mg/d of tiopronin, both in divided doses. Unfortunately, both have drawbacks of possible leukopenia, aplastic anemia, proteinuria, and hepatotoxicity, with tiopronin tolerated slightly better.[24]

For infection or struvite stones, the key to treatment is retrieval of the stone because bacteria can live uninhibited by antibiotics in the interior of the stone. Urine culture and targeted antibiotics are key as well as referral to urology for percutaneous nephrolithotomy.[15] When retrieval is not possible, medical therapy with urease inhibitor acetohydroxamic acid is indicated. Three randomized controlled trials have shown proved decrease in growth of stones using this medication. Use of this drug is complicated by its high side-effect profile, including significant gastrointestinal upset[24] (**Table 2**).

POTENTIAL COMPLICATIONS

The main complications of renal stones are pyonephrosis (infected urine behind an obstructing stone) and hydronephrosis (complete blockage of the ureter with

Table 2
Dietary and Pharmacologic Intervention

Type of Stone	Target Urinary pH	Recommended Diet	Pharmaceuticals/Supplements to Consider	Drugs to Avoid
Calcium	Alkaline	Low in animal protein, high in potassium-rich fruits/vegetables; DASH diet	Thiazides, potassium citrate, allopurinol	Loop diuretics, acetazolamide, topiramate, zonisamide
Uric acid	Alkaline	Low in purine-containing foods	Allopurinol, potassium citrate	Probenecid, ammonium acid laxatives
Cystine	Alkaline	Low in animal protein, high in potassium-rich fruits/vegetables	Potassium citrate, D-penicillamine, tiopronin	—
Struvite	Alkaline	Low in animal protein, high in potassium-rich fruits/vegetables	Targeted antibiotics, Acetohydroxamic acid	—

Legent

subsequent urine collection). Both of these can cause significant morbidity. Pyonephrosis requires immediate drainage of the obstructed kidney, which can be accomplished either percutaneously or with a renal stent. Hydronephrosis also requires drainage in a similar manner. Hydronephrosis may be silent, however. The stone may become impacted in the ureter and then become covered with urothelium. This causes a more gradual collection of urine and the kidney eventually becomes atrophic and nonfunctioning. Surprisingly, this may cause little to no pain due to the gradual nature of the buildup.[28]

Another concerning complication may be increased risk of chronic kidney disease (CKD). One study found an increased risk in men with CKD: 15.21% had a history of renal stones versus 11.4% without. The difference was higher in women: 23.18% with versus 13.48% without renal stones.[29] The study did not state if there were other complications related to the treatment of the stone—just whether a history of stones was present.

NEPHROLOGY CONSULTATION/REFERRAL

Although urology is the mainstay in referral for acute surgical management of nephrolithiasis, referring to nephrology may be needed at times for the sequela and further management of recurrence of nephrolithiasis. There is an increased risk for CKD in patients with history of multiple symptomatic kidney stones shown in recent population studies. Stone formers have been seen, in a population-based historical cohort study, to be at increased risk of CKD, even when controlled for the usual causes of diabetes, hypertension, or obesity. The risk for clinical CKD was 50% to 65% greater in stone formers.[26] Although nephrolithiasis is an infrequent cause of kidney failure, struvite (infection) stones have been associated with an increased risk of acute kidney failure or CKD.[15]

Patients with recurrent nephrolithiasis should be referred to nephrology for a detailed evaluation of metabolic factors to determine preventable causes of the stones as well as aiming at promoting resolution of any existing stones. Also, consideration should be given to referral to a nephrologist when treating patients who have a family history of renal calculi along with inflammatory bowel disease, frequent UTIs, or a history of nephrocalcinosis, which is found most frequently incidentally while imaging in the quest for diagnosis of stones.[15,18]

SUMMARY

Nephrolithiasis or kidney stones is the second most common CKD, affecting 12% of all people. Early recognition and treatment of this condition are important to prevent complications that can occur with delayed treatment. Furthermore, increasing prevalence of this disease underlines the importance of correctly diagnosing the causative factors, thereby affecting prevention of recurrence.

ACKNOWLEDGMENTS

(**Tables 1, 2**) and (**Boxes 1, 2**) were created by Lorena Clare Bishop, a student at Belhaven University.

DISCLOSURE

The authors have nothing to disclose.

REFERENCES

1. Worcester EM, Coe FL. Nephrolithiasis. Prim Care 2008;35(2):369.
2. William S. Medical definition of nephrolithiasis. MedicineNet 2018.
3. Tefekli A, Cezayirli F. The history of urinary stones: In parallel with civilization. ScientificWorldJournal 2013;2013:423964.
4. Pawar AS, Thongprayoon C, Cheungpasitporn W, et al. Incidence and characteristics of kidney stones in patients with horseshoe kidney: A systematic review and meta-analysis. Urol Ann 2018;10(1):87–93.
5. Scales CD, Smith AC, Hanley JM, et al. Prevalence of kidney stones in the United States. Eur Urol 2012;62(1):160–5.
6. Wein A, Kavoussi L, Partin A, et al. Campbell-walsh urology. Philadelphia: Elsevier; 2015.
7. Bansal AD, Hui J, Goldfarb DS. Asymptomatic nephrolithiasis detected by ultrasound. Clin J Am Soc Nephrol 2009;4(3):680.
8. Mayans L. Nephrolithiasis. Prim Care 2019;46(2):203–12.
9. Hall P. Nephrolithiasis: treatment, causes, and prevention. Cleve Clin J Med 2009; 76(10):583.
10. Gottlieb M, Long B, Koyfman A. The evaluation and management of urolithiasis in the ED: A review of the literature. Am J Emerg Med 2018;36(4):699–706.
11. Teichman J. Clinical practice. Acute renal colic from ureteral calculus. N Engl J Med 2004;350(7):684–93.
12. Li J, Kennedy D, Levine M, et al. Absent hematuria and expensive computerized tomography: case characteristics of emergency urolithiasis. J Urol 2001;165(3): 782–4.
13. Curhan G, Aronson M, Preminger G. Diagnosis and acute management of suspected nephrolithiasis in adults. 2019. Available at: www.uptodate.com. Accessed October 1, 2019.
14. Krambeck AE, Lieske JC, Li X, et al. Effect of age on the clinical presentation of incident symptomatic urolithiasis in the general population. J Urol 2013;189(1): 158–64.
15. Pfau A, Knauf F. Update on nephrolithiasis: core curriculum 2016. Am J Kidney Dis 2016;58(6):973–85.
16. Chandrashekar KB, Fulop T, Juncos LA. Medical management and prevention of nephrolithiasis. Am J Med 2012;125(4):344–7.
17. Izzedine H, Lescure FX, Bonnet F. HIV medication-based urolithiasis. Clin Kidney J 2017;7(2):121–6.
18. Paige NM, Nagami GT. The top 10 things nephrologists wish every primary care physician knew. Mayo Clin Proc 2009;84(2):180–6.
19. Torricelli FC, De S, Liu X, et al. Can 24-hour urine stone risk profiles predict urinary stone composition? J Endourol 2014;28(6):735–8.
20. Qaseem A, Dallas P, Forciea MA, et al. Dietary and pharmacologic management to prevent recurrent nephrolithiasis in adults: a clinical Practice guideline from the american college of physicians. Ann Intern Med 2014;161(9):659–67.
21. S. 2680 (115th): Opioid crisis response act of 2018.
22. Pathan SA, Mitra B, Cameron PA. A systematic review and meta-analysis comparing the efficacy of nonsteroidal anti-inflammatory drugs, opioids, and paracetamol in the treatment of acute renal colic. Eur Urol 2018;73(4):583–95.
23. Garcia-Perdomo HA, Echeverria-Garcia F, Lopez H, et al. Pharmacologic interventions to treat renal colic pain in acute stone episodes: systematic review and meta-analysis. Prog Urol 2017;27(12):654–65.

24. Zisman AL. Effectiveness of treatment modalities on kidney stone recurrence. Clin J Am Soc Nephrol 2017;12(10):1699–708.
25. Alelign T, Petros B. Kidney stone disease: an update on current concepts. Adv Urol 2018;2018:12. Article ID 3068365.
26. Rule AD, Krambeck AE, Lieske JC. Chronic kidney disease in kidney stone formers. Clin J Am Soc Nephrol 2011;6(8):2069–75.
27. Matlaga BR, Shah OD, Assimos DG. Drug-induced urinary calculi. Rev Urol 2003; 5(4):227–31.
28. Kellerman R, Rakel D. Conn's current therapy. Philadelphia: Elsevier; 2019.
29. Shoag J, Halpern J, Goldfarb DS, et al. Risk of chronic and end stage kidney disease in patients with nephrolithiasis. J Urol 2014;192(5):1440–5.

Autosomal Dominant Polycystic Kidney Disease

Parvathi Perumareddi, DO*, Darin P. Trelka, MD, PhD

KEYWORDS

- Polycystic kidney disease • End-stage renal disease • Dialysis • Transplant
- Secondary hypertension • Berry aneurysm • Hematuria • Liver cysts

KEY POINTS

- ADPKD is a genetic disease characterized by early cystic development in the kidneys and liver resulting in enlarged kidneys and liver.
- One of the most common presentations is early onset hypertension.
- Risk factor modification is vital but V2 receptor antagonists may play a role.
- The course of disease is variable but many individuals progress to ESRD eventually requiring renal transplant.

INTRODUCTION

Autosomal dominant polycystic kidney disease (ADPKD) is one of the most common hereditary disorders overall and is the most common of the renal cystic diseases.[1] AKPKD is a genetic disorder characterized by the formation of multiple renal cysts, kidney enlargement, symptoms related to distorted structure and abnormal function, and ultimately renal dysfunction.[2]

Extrarenal effects can occur in various other sites affecting organs, such as the liver, brain, and pancreas, thus making this a systemic condition whose damage is irreversible.[2]

The pathologic course of ADPKD is gradual and progressive often resulting in destruction of the renal parenchyma and leading to end-stage renal failure by age 60 years in up to one-half of patients.[3]

Although the cysts may be detectable as early as in utero, their growth in size and quantity is slow over years such that clinical symptoms are usually not apparent until the third or fourth decades,[4] making the diagnosis unobtrusive. Since the cysts affect a small number of nephrons and a compensatory mechanism exists such that renal function is preserved for decades, this diagnosis is often not readily apparent early on.[2]

Florida Atlantic University, Schmidt College of Medicine, 777 Glades Road, Boca Raton, FL 33431, USA
* Corresponding author. Florida Atlantic University, Schmidt College of Medicine, 777 Glades Road, ME-104, Boca Raton, FL 33431, USA
E-mail address: pperumar@health.fau.edu

Prim Care Clin Office Pract 47 (2020) 673–689
https://doi.org/10.1016/j.pop.2020.08.010
0095-4543/20/© 2020 Elsevier Inc. All rights reserved.

Laboratory values related to renal function do not decline until after damage has occurred. Occasionally, the diagnosis is made incidentally through imaging or laboratory work for other unrelated symptoms or conditions or by the onset of early hypertension, one of the most prominent clues for ADPKD.[5]

Although most patients progress to end-stage renal disease (ESRD) ultimately requiring renal replacement, not all do, and the spectrum of renal impact can be wide or often variable.[6]

Treatment has been historically supportive in nature, focusing mostly on management of symptoms and associated conditions but, recently, targeted treatments are being investigated based on the elucidation of specific pathophysiologic mechanisms. Studies have been underway to ascertain treatments that may slow the progression of this disease, because currently there is no known cure.

Because patients typically have hypertension and sometimes other common symptoms, primary care physicians need to be familiar with the presentation of ADPKD and resposit it within their differential diagnoses list early on, to recognize and refer to Nephrology for immediate treatment and surveillance, because early intervention is crucial to initiating valuable treatment, which can affect quality of life sooner.

INCIDENCE/PREVALENCE

Globally, there are approximately 12 million people with ADPKD. In the United States, the number of individuals with ADPKD is estimated at 600,000 people or 1 in 500 to 1 in 1000 live births.[7]

The penetrance is heterogenous, and distribution is almost equal among women and men with each offspring possessing a 50% chance of inheriting the genetic mutation and the disease.[2] The two gene sites associated with mutations in ADPKD are PKD1 and PKD2. The prevalence, age at occurrence, and severity are significantly different between the two.[8] PKD1 constitutes approximately 85% of cases, and PKD2 makes up the remainder or 15%.[9] Of the two types, ADPKD1 has an earlier onset and a more severe course with the mean age of ESRD occurring at 53 years, whereas ADPKD2 tends to occur later and is less severe with a mean age of ESRD occurring at 74 years.[8]

PATHOGENESIS/PATHOPHYSIOLOGY

Most commonly, ADPKD is caused by mutations in the PKD1 or PKD2 genes, which encode polycystin 1 (PC1)[10] and polycystin 2 (PC2) proteins,[11] respectively. The PC1 and PC2 proteins are integral membrane proteins of the primary cilia of renal tubule epithelial cells.[10] PC1 and PC2 are functionally and structurally related proteins that form heterodimeric complexes with one another through interactions between their cytoplasmic C-terminal domains to regulate intracellular calcium and cyclic adenosine monophosphate (cAMP), although the exact functions of this complex have yet to be fully elucidated.[10–13] Cystogenesis is thought to result from a "two-hit" model wherein the first hit is the aforementioned "recessive" germline mutation in one of the polycystin genes, followed by the acquisition of a second somatic mutation, which inactivates the remaining normal polycystin allele.[11,13] A "third hit" has been postulated, representing toxic or ischemic insult to the affected kidney(s), which may trigger a "repair response."[13] This was posited in experimental mouse models wherein mutations in both the PKD1 genes alone did not result in cystogenesis for several months; and, because the "second hit" likely does not occur until after maturation of the kidneys, the third hit of damage and subsequent repair are also hypothesized to be required in humans.[13] Furthermore, Torres and colleagues[13] reported

that, in their mouse model, cystogenesis was dependent on formation of calcium oxalate and calcium phosphate crystals in kidney tubule lumena of mice and that citrate treatment, as a chelator of calcium, reduced both crystal formation and
cystogenesis, although the mechanism(s) of cystogenesis have yet to be completely
described.[11]

CYSTOGENESIS

Progressive nephron structural perturbation and functional loss due to cystogenesis is
clinically silent for the first few decades of life, although it can begin during fetal development.[10] The early clinical silence is likely due to compensatory hyperfiltration by the
remaining intact nephrons.[10] The enlargement of renal cysts has been described to
result from both increased hyperfiltration in the lumen of the nascent cyst as well as
alterations in tubular epithelial cell polarity, increased extracellular matrix production,
and mitogenic response.[10,11] The aforementioned alterations are thought to occur in
tandem with alterations in the microvasculature and functioning nephrons surrounding
nascent cysts, which begin to become extrinsically compressed and results in structural and spatial separation of the cysts, which then continue to enlarge by transepi-
thelial fluid shifts.[10] The cysts enlarge and increase in number over time to a critical
point; the impairment progresses to kidney failure.[12] The physical compression on
the vessels added to the release of inflammatory substances results in fibrosis and
inflammation. See **Fig. 1**.[10,11]

PKD1 and PKD2 are expressed throughout the body and work in conjunction with
one another in forming the morphology of the epithelial cells, with much concentration
focused on their function in the kidney, liver, and vascular smooth muscle cells.

One of the earlier dysfunctions that occurs is a decrease in urine-concentrating ability, but the reason is unknown. Increased vasopressin levels are thought to occur as a
compensatory mechanism for the reduced concentrating ability and has been

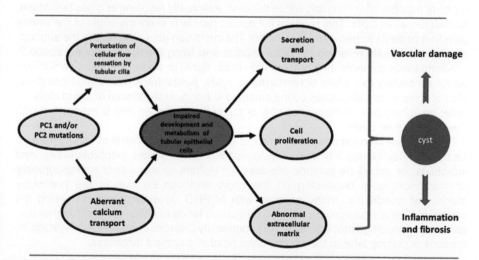

Fig. 1. Postulated pathogenesis of cysts in ADPKD. (*Data from* Gimpel C, Bergmann C, Bockenhauer D, et al. International consensus statement on the diagnosis and management of
autosomal dominant polycystic kidney disease in children and young people. Nat Rev.
2019;15:713–26; and Salvadori M, Tsalouchos A. New therapies targeting cystogenesis in
autosomal polycystic kidney disease. EMJ Nephrol. 2017;5(1):102–11.)

postulated as a contributing factor to the formation of the kidney cysts, renal functional decline, and the development of hypertension.

CLINICAL PRESENTATION

Patients with ADPKD are often asymptomatic early in life with symptoms first appearing around the fourth decade.[9] Some symptoms develop as a result of actual expansion, compression, or rupture of the cysts, whereas other symptoms occur due to physiologic dysfunction.[2]

Suspicion for and subsequent diagnosis of ADPKD may occur in several scenarios. The diagnosis is often made incidentally or in the process of work ups for other conditions or laboratory abnormalities, but the most common initial symptom complaint is pain, abdominal, back, or flank, which is present in most patients.[1] Also, as eluded to previously, many patients develop hypertension. Therefore, a discovery of high blood pressure in a younger patient may be the herald of a diagnosis of ADPKD.[14]

Below are the findings commonly associated with ADPKD that should raise suspicion for the consideration of the diagnosis[9]:

- Early onset hypertension
- Hematuria
- Pain in abdomen, flank, or back
- Palpable abdominal/flank masses[15]
- Renal insufficiency or progressive declining renal function
- Family history of ADPKD

The is delay in symptomology is thought to result from compensatory mechanisms that involve hyperfiltration resulting in preservation of aggregate glomerular filtration rate, until after at least the third or fourth decade of life when renal dysfunction becomes more evident with a reduction of 4.4 to 5.9 mL per minute per year.[12]

The cysts are linked with excessive angiogenesis,[16] which, with trauma, can rupture, thus causing bleeding within the cyst, eventually resulting in gross hematuria, sometimes even clots. This process if it occurs rapidly is likely the origin of the severe pain that patients sometimes experience. The cysts can also rupture into the subcapsular compartment invading the renal capsule and filling the retroperitoneal space.[17]

Alternatively, patients may present with back, flank, or abdominal pain,[1] which can occur secondary to rupture of hemorrhagic cysts, actual frank obstruction/compression of surrounding structures by the enlarged kidneys, or by release of blood clots. Of note, an aching pain or heaviness may occur in the abdomen and is associated with the multiple liver cysts.

Patients may also experience symptoms of renal colic as a result of urinary tract infections (UTIs), kidney infections (pyelonephritis), renal stones (nephrolithiasis), cyst infections, or actual perinephric abscesses.[6] Hematuria can occur microscopically or macroscopically depending on the origin and can be due to the previously mentioned conditions. Many patients with ADPKD develop hematuria during the course of their disease progression. Hypertension tends to occur early with higher corresponding readings that are initially predominantly diastolic increases with systolic increases occurring later in the course once renal impairment advances.

DIAGNOSIS
History

If ADPKD is suspected, the following history can be helpful in narrowing the differential[1]:

- Family history of ADPKD
- History of hypertension, diabetes, or cardiovascular disease
- Presence of multiorgan disease
- History of recurrent UTIs or current UTIs
- Past glomerular disease
- Medication history, especially nonsteroidal anti-inflammatory drugs (NSAIDs) or other nephrotoxic drugs

Physical Examination

A focused physical examination may reveal abnormalities[9] related to either renal dysfunction or as a direct result from the space occupied by the cysts and renal enlargement.

The following components of the physical examination are important to perform:

- Blood pressure (including history readings)
- Cardiovascular examination → mitral valve prolapse
- Abdominal examination → palpable mass
- Lower extremity examination → edema
- Abdominal auscultation → renal bruit

Laboratory Testing

Routine laboratory testing is performed as for other conditions of chronic kidney disease and typically consists of:

- Chemistry profile (BMP)
- Serum calcium
- Serum phosphorus
- Urinalysis
- Urine culture
- Uric acid
- Intact PTH
- CBC

Genetic Testing

Genetic testing is not widely used as a method of diagnosis of ADPKD, but it can be useful in preconception counseling. For family members of a patient with ADPKD, current practice does not routinely use genetic testing for confirmation, but rather utilizes imaging, which is useful for early detection in these cases.[9]

Imaging Criteria

Diagnosis of ADPKD is achieved using imaging, with ultrasound being the preferred modality due to its ease of accessibility, lower cost, and lack of radiation risks. However, the efficacy of renal ultrasound in diagnosis of ADPKD is limited to the size of the nascent cysts, as small cysts (less than 1 cm) may be difficult to visualize.[6]

Axial computed tomography (CT) and MRI are more sensitive, approaching 100% in detecting cysts with smaller diameters, 2 to 3 mm, and should be considered if ultrasound results are equivocal; this may also be the case in patients who are obese and in younger patients known to have risk factors.[18] In general, CT and MRI are not used routinely for initial diagnosis. MRI, however, is utilized in monitoring disease progression, treatment efficacy, or prognosis once a diagnosis is made and treatment initiated.[18]

High-definition ultrasound is 1 method that can be useful if available and may provide more accurate findings, but its utility depends on the expertise of the sonographer and may not easily be accessible. If it is available, however, it can be particularly useful in the identification of smaller cysts.[18]

Unified ultrasonographic criteria were established by Ravine and colleagues[19] for diagnosis of ADPKD based on age, family history, and risk status, as shown in **Table 1**.[20]

It should be noted that imaging-based diagnosis was developed on the presumption of 50% positive family history and in age-related categories; therefore, for those who do not have a family history, which constitutes 10% to 25% of patients, the imaging criteria would not be applicable.[19,20]

DISEASE PROGRESSION

Many manifestations of ADPKD exist, some presenting as chronic conditions and others that may arise acutely, either systemically or within the urinary tract.

Hypertension often develops in the fourth decade, but signs such as proteinuria and chronic pain develop later.[17] Hematuria can occur throughout the course as can the signs/symptoms of cystic rupture.[9]

Cyst infection and stones tend to occur after the age of 30 years (**Fig. 2**).

Over time, the kidneys grow in size and volume due to continuous development of cysts. Despite this growth, the decrease in glomerular filtration rate (GFR) occurs insidiously and sometimes stabilizes. This maintenance in function is due to the compensatory hyperfiltration by the remaining nephrons.[2] Because of this, the GFR is an inaccurate measure of progression of disease.[20]

Patients with PKD1 defects tend to have more cysts and larger kidneys as a result, with most progressing to kidney failure before age 70 years.[1] However, patients with PKD2 have a less severe course such that their renal function remains stable. Regardless of general trends, it is worthwhile noting that there is variability in symptom course and progression even within each type of ADPKD.

Because renal function, as measured by serum creatinine and estimate GFR, cannot accurately predict progression of disease as is the case in typical chronic kidney disease, other methods to determine progression have been investigated.[20]

A landmark study conducted at the Mayo Clinic, Consortium for Radiologic Imaging Studies of Polycystic Kidney Disease (CRISP), was established in 2001 and

Table 1
Unified Ravine criteria for diagnosis of ADPKD

Age (y)	Positive Family History	Positive Predictive Value
15–29	At least 3 cysts in one or both kidneys	100
30–39	At least 3 cysts in one or both kidneys	100
40–59	At least 2 cysts in each kidney	100
>60	At least 4 cysts in each kidney	100

Data from Ravine D, Sheffield LJ, Danks DM, et al. Evaluation of ultrasonographic diagnostic criteria for autosomal dominant polycystic kidney disease. The Lancet. 1994;343(8901):824–7; and Pei Y, Obaji J, Dupuis A, et al. Unified criteria for ultrasonographic diagnosis of ADPKD. J Am Soc Nephrol. 2009; 20(1):205–12.

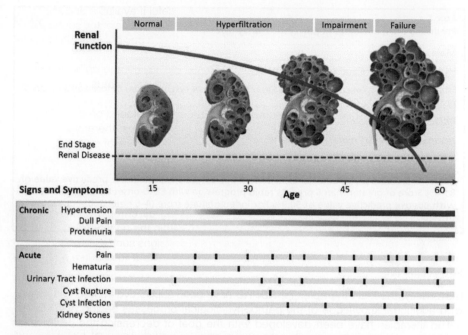

Fig. 2. Typical disease progression in ADPKD. (*Courtesy of* Otsuka Pharmaceutical Development and Commercialization Inc, Rockville, MD.)

has been ongoing to determine whether imaging modalities could provide accurate and reproducible assessment of the progression of renal disease inADPKD.[20]

The outcomes confirmed that increase in total kidney volume (TKV), which occurs initially, is a result of the increase in the volume of renal cysts and that a significant inverse relationship exists between the increase in cyst and kidney volume versus the decline in the estimated GFR (eGFR). The study also determined the association between TKV and other associated pathophysiological abnormalities, such as hypertension, hematuria, proteinuria, microalbuminuria, and longitudinal decline in kidney function.[20]

Hypertension is one of the most common presenting signs in ADPKD. Although the disease is progressive, if one develops hypertension at a relatively younger age, this is also related to a more rapid decline in renal function.[21,22]

Several other factors are associated with faster disease progression including[21,22]:

- PKD1 mutation
- Early age at diagnosis
- Male gender
- Early decrease in GFR
- Early onset of hypertension
- High TKV (Mayo classification 1C-1E)
- Multiple pregnancies (3 or more)

The predicting renal outcomes in polycystic kidney disease (PROPKD) is a tool that uses factors, such as genetics and clinical factors to provide stratification of the risks of decline in ADPKD and with subsequent advancement to ESRD[22] (**Box 1**).

Box 1
Predicting renal outcomes in polycystic kidney disease

Male sex: 1 point

Hypertension before age 35 years: 2 points

First urologic event (microscopic hematuria, flank pain or cyst infection) before age 35 years: 2 points

PKD2 mutation: 0 points

Nontruncating PKD1 mutation: 2 points

Truncating PKD1 mutation: 4 points

Score ≤3 excludes progression to ESRD before age 60 years with negative predictive value of 81.4%.Score of greater than 6 predicts rapid progression with ESRD onset before age 60 years with positive predictive value of 90.9%.For indeterminate score (4–6 points), the prognosis is unclear.[22]

SURVEILLANCE

Historically, the main therapies for ADPKD have been supportive in nature; however, with additional knowledge of the pathophysiological processes behind ADPKD, targeted therapies have been developed with the goal of decreasing the proliferation of kidney cysts as well as decelerating the decline in renal function. Risk factor modification remains a critical treatment goal as cardiovascular disease remains the most common cause of mortality in patients with ADPKD.

There have been several randomized controlled trials, some of which have resulted in clinically useful diagnostic modalities and therapies. **Fig. 3** illustrates the various landmark trials in ADPKD conducted over the past 3 decades.

Initial studies revealed that arginine vasopressin-mediated cAMP is a catalyst in the proliferation of renal cysts and accumulation of cyst fluid.[6] Rodent studies revealed

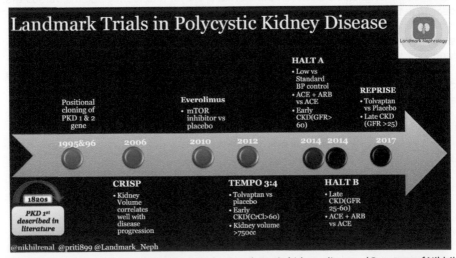

Fig. 3. Landmark trials in autosomal dominant polycystic kidney disease. (*Courtesy of* Nikhil Agrawal, LandmarkNephrology.com, Twitter @landmark_neph.)

that several factors reduced the growth of cysts, namely, an increase in water intake, which resulted in inhibition of vasopressin, genetic elimination of vasopressin, and antagonism of vasopressin V2 receptor. The latter of these was studied in human subjects with ADPKD, which was in the TEMP 3:4 study. In this RCT, 1445 patients with ADPKD who were at risk for progression were treated with tolvaptan (a V2 receptor antagonist), which revealed a decrease in TKV over 3 years in the study with the initial year showing the greatest effects.

Renal functional decline was the secondary endpoint in the study and also revealed significant results. The untoward effects that occurred were related to aquaretic side effects, polyuria, polydipsia, and nocturia.[6] Notably, liver enzyme tests were found to be increased. Although the transaminase levels were significantly high, there were no cases of liver failure. However, for safety reasons, an official recommendation for monitoring was issued.[6]

After the US Food and Drug Administration requested additional information determining the efficacy and safety of tolvaptan in patients with advanced ADPKD, the Replicating Evidence of Preserved Renal Function: An Investigation of Tolvaptan Safety and Efficacy (REPRISE) was created.[6,23]

Unlike the TEMPO 3:4 trial, patients enrolled in the REPRISE trial were those with more advanced disease. This trial revealed a reduction in decline of eGFR in the first year in patients who were given tolvaptan. The effect was limited to those who were younger than 55 years but was similar to that of renin-angiotensinogen-aldosterone inhibitors.[6]

Although there is no official consensus in whom and when therapy with tolvaptan should be given, general practices includes[14,17,23,24]:

- Age less than 55 years
- Chronic kidney disease stage 1-3a
    (eGFR > or = 45 mL/min per 1.73 m^2)
- High risk measured by available risk scores
    (Mayo classification of 1C, 1D, or 1E, TKV >750 mL, or PROPKD score >6)
- History of decline in eGFR
    (>or = 5 mL/min per 1.73 m^2 in 1 year or at least 2.5 mL/min per 1.73 m^2/year
    for 5 years)

CLINICAL MANIFESTATIONS/COMPLICATIONS AND MANAGEMENT

Various renal and extrarenal manifestations are associated with ADPKD and can cause symptoms affecting daily life, thus requiring treatment.

Table 2 illustrates some of the most common associated conditions.

Hypertension

Hypertension is known to develop in most patients with ADPKD (~60%) before decline in renal function.[9] It typically commences in the 30s and, in this earlier age range, the prominent abnormality tends to be diastolic increase, whereas, after the 50s, the dysfunction occurs predominantly in systolic readings.

There are several thoughts as to why hypertension arises in patients with ADPKD. One mechanism is the activation of the renin-angiotensin-aldosterone (RAAS) system, which is potentially caused by the cysts physically compressing the vasculature resulting in ischemia.[21,25]

The other proposed mechanisms involve vascular dysfunction and increased sympathetic tone.[21,25]

Table 2
Most common associations with ADPKD

Manifestation	Occurrence	Notes
Hypertension	50%–70%	Treat with ACE-I or ARB
Abdominal/flank pain	Up to 60%	Avoid NSAIDs, acetaminophen
Nephrolithiasis	20%–35%	Uric acid, calcium oxalate Copious fluids, ESWL
Cyst hemorrhage	Up to 60%	Rest, spontaneous resolution
Urinary tract infection	30%–50%	Fluoroquinolones
Polycystic liver	Up to 80%	Debulking, drainage
Intracranial aneurysm	20%–27% in those with positive family history; 9% without such family history	Treat if symptomatic
Arachnoid cysts	8%–12%	
Mitral valve prolapse	~25%	Screen if symptomatic (palpitations) Beta blockers
Pericardial effusion	Up to 35%	Screen if symptomatic
Pancreatic cysts	~10%	No screening recommended
Diverticulosis	20%–25% in ESRD	No screening recommended
Bronchiectasis	Up to 37%	No screening recommended
Seminal vesicle cysts	Up to 40%	No correlation to semen abnormalities
Male infertility	Association	Abnormal semen parameters

Abbreviations: ACE-I, angiotensin-converting enzyme inhibitor; ARB, angiotensin receptor blockers; ESWL, extracorporeal shock wave lithotripsy.
Adapted from Chebib FT, Torres VE. Autosomal polycystic kidney disease: core curriculum 2016. Am J Kidney Dis. 2016;67(5):800; with permission.

Treatment of hypertension remains the cornerstone of management of ADPKD for all patients.

The Halt Progression of Polycystic Kidney Disease (HALT-PKD) study is a randomized, double-blind, placebo-controlled clinical trial that was conducted between 2006 and 2014 at multicenters of 2 concurrent studies formulated to assess the efficacy of RAAS inhibition on the decline in renal function and progression of cystic disease.[17]

Study arm A investigated treatment in patients with early ADPKD with a standard versus intensive blood pressure goal for both arms (120–130/70–80 mm Hg versus 95–110/60–75 mm Hg). There was a proven decrease in TKV as well as reductions in left ventricular mass, proteinuria, and renal vascular resistance in the more intensive blood pressure group versus the standard one.[25]

The other arm of the HALT-PKD study involved treating patients with moderate ADPKD with both angiotensin-converting enzyme inhibitors (ACE-Is) and angiotensin II receptor blockers (ARBs) to standard blood pressure target goal; however, no benefit was shown with combination therapy.

There were no differences, however, between the groups on monotherapy with ACE-I versus dual therapy with ACE-Is and ARBs.[23,25] Treatment with ACE-Is or ARBs is recommended as first-line with a goal of less than or equal to 110/75 mm Hg for patients aged 18 to 50 years with preserved eGFR (greater than or equal to 60 mL/min).[17,24]

Ambulatory blood pressure recording is found to be the most ideal for monitoring. As in other disease states, optimal blood pressure control is essential in slowing the progression of renal functional decline. Once a patient reaches ESRD, they are more prone to hyperkalemia, particularly when taking ACE-Is or ARBs; thus, interval monitoring of electrolytes is warranted. Most patients with ADPKD require at least 2 antihypertensives to achieve goal blood pressure and, although there is no consensus on an exact blood pressure goal, there is evidence that lower blood pressure preserves nephrons, therefore, a suggested target B/P is 130/80 mmHg.[6]

CYSTIC INFECTION AND HEMORRHAGE

Infections are relatively uncommon but, when they do occur, they can be difficult to manage because they must be treated with antibiotics that penetrate the inner cavity of the cysts, such as fluoroquinolones and trimethoprim-sulfamethoxazole. If the antibiotics fail to treat the cystic masses, CT-guided aspiration may be performed. If the cysts are larger (>5 cm), treatment with both antibiotics and drainage tends to be more effective.[26]

Cyst hemorrhage is a common occurrence but tends to resolve spontaneously in less than a week with rest[17]; however, any other potential malignant etiologies must be eliminated if it persists.

CARDIOVASCULAR DISEASE

Since hypertension occurs at a younger age in patients with ADPKD and is often accompanied by left ventricular hypertrophy and occasionally valvular dysfunction, cardiovascular disease is the most common cause of death.[27] It is thought that statins may have a positive effect on regression of renal cyst size due to pleomorphic effects,[2,6] but no studies have concluded a specific unique target goal for low-density lipoprotein in ADPKD. Risk factor modification of lipid levels as dictated for chronic kidney disease (CKD) or cardiovascular disease (CVD) is indicated.

CEREBRAL ANEURYSM

Saccular berry aneurysms occur in a small percentage of patients (approximately 5%–10%), with ruptures occurring at younger ages compared with those without ADPKD.[27,28]

However, because this condition is potentially fatal, it must be considered in all patients with ADPKD. Regardless, the risk of rupture is relatively low.[9] Although routine screening is not recommended, certain settings call for imaging to rule out an intracranial bleed. **Table 3** lists criteria that indicate the necessity for aneurysm screening.[28]

HEPATIC CYSTS

Liver cysts concomitantly develop with the renal cysts and occur in 80% to 90% of patients after age 35 years.[6]

In addition to the usual/expected propensity for patients with ADPKD to develop extrarenal cysts, certain additional risk factors also influence the development of hepatic cysts:

- Hormone replacement therapy
- Oral contraceptive therapy
- Multiple pregnancies

The above implying hormonal influence in women.[6]

Table 3	
General criteria for aneurysm screening	
Family history of intracranial aneurysm or ICH	
Previous history of intracranial aneurysm rupture	
CNS symptoms:	New onset severe headache Nausea and vomiting Seizures Loss of consciousness Photophobia Transient ischemic attack
Before major surgery: eg, renal transplant	
Initiation of long-term anticoagulation	
High-risk occupation:	Pilot Bus drivers
Patient anxiety or concern after education	

Abbreviations: ICH, intracranial hemorrhage.
Data from Hughes PDV, Becker GJ. Screening for intracranial aneurysms in autosomal polycystic kidney disease. Nephrology 2003;8(4):163–70.

When the hepatic cysts become large, although they do not cause disruption of actual liver function (increased transaminase levels), symptoms occur that can interfere with a patient's quality of life including[9]:

- Abdominal pain
- Abdominal distention
- Early satiety
- Dyspnea

The dyspnea occurring as a result of pressure on the diaphragm. Interventions are variable depending on patient symptoms and impact on quality of life and range from narcotics for pain to cyst fenestration to hepatectomy. It is important to note that cysts may recur with resultant massive enlargement of the liver.[29,30]

Hepatic transplantation is the only curative treatment and, although rarely performed, it may be considered once the liver becomes so enlarged causing unbearable symptoms or if portal hypertension develops.[29,30]

As with renal colic, it is important to avoid the use of NSAIDs as they can contribute to worsening renal function.

OTHER CONSIDERATIONS

- If diagnosis of ADPKD is uncertain, ensure diagnosis of renal cell carcinoma is eliminated
- Medications used to treat pain or other conditions pose challenges as many medications are eliminated renally and should be avoided. For example, NSAIDs should not be recommended. There are no medications that can be safely given for osteoporosis secondary to route of elimination. Also, administration of vitamin D and calcium present issues secondary to hypercalcemia in ESRD
- Anemia is often present as expected in CKD and therefore typical symptoms may include fatigue and pallor
- Because there is a heterogenous penetrance, extensive education and genetic counseling/testing should be offered to patients and family members

ADDITIONAL INTERVENTIONS

Various lifestyle modifications are recommended to mitigate the decline in renal function and associated cardiovascular risk factors. Patient education in these areas is important as these are actions they can take to potentially reduce some of the negative consequences of this disease.

Hydration

There are ongoing studies established to determine the effect of water consumption on ADPKD,[6] particularly because of the role of vasopressin in the potential attenuation of cyst growth; however, there has been no definitive correlative effect to date, although from a physiologic standpoint reduction in cyst growth seems plausible with intake of copious fluids. However, because of the increased incidence of kidney stones, it is often recommended that patients with ADPKD consume upward of 3 L of water/day to prevent formation of stones.[6]

Sodium Intake

Consuming high amounts of dietary sodium is known to increase blood pressure as well as being a risk factor for cardiovascular disease. Studies have been conducted focusing on the effect of dietary sodium levels in patients with ADPKD, finding sodium excretion to be associated with a sharper decline in eGFR and increased risk of kidney enlargement in analysis of the HALT-PKD study.[30] There is thought also that dietary sodium results in progression of ADPKD because of vasopressin stimulation.[31]

The general recommendation based on these findings is for patients to limit sodium intake to a maximum of 2.3 to 3 g/d, although even less may be beneficial as is the case with hypertension.[9]

Tobacco Use

It has been shown in patients with ADPKD that smoking has a detrimental effect as it does in cardiovascular disease and other conditions. It is associated with risk of ESRD and faster progression of disease.[32] Vasopressin secretion is increased with smoking and may be the reason for disease progression as well as an increased risk of intracranial aneurysm rupture.[2] Smoking cessation and/or abstinence should be strongly encouraged.

Activity

Although there is no specific recommendation for exercise levels or amounts, it has been shown that there is an association between obesity and reduced renal function (eGFR and greater percent change in TKV).[32]

The Kidney Disease: Improving Global Outcomes has suggested a recommendation for 30 min of moderate exercise on at least 5 days per week for patients with CKD.[32]

Weight-bearing exercises are also helpful for osteoporosis, which can occur in patients with CKD and as above, can be challenging to treat.

Diet

Since there have been no dedicated studies on the role of specific dietary interventions in relation to regression or management of ADPKD that have proven beneficial, findings from non- ADPKD have been extrapolated to serve as general recommendations.

For prevention of cardiovascular mortality, there are 2 studies that have shown a consistent proven benefit, namely Dietary Approaches to Stop Hypertension and PREDIMED.[31]

Of note, intermittent fasting and calorie reduction are being studied.

It is unknown whether any of these interventions reduce renal functional decline; however, since cardiovascular disease is the most common cause of death in patients with ADPKD, these remain worthwhile modifications to prevent or reduce CVD.

END-STAGE RENAL DISEASE

The optimal treatment of ESRD in patients with ADPKD is kidney transplantation,[33] with a living donor being the preferred. The decision for timing of transplantation is not based on a specific level of renal failure but often dictated by a combination of renal function and presence of related symptoms that are negatively affecting the patient's quality of life on an individual basis. Evaluation for transplant potential along with work up should be conducted early and may eliminate the need for dialysis, which can be detrimental over time; however, the patient should be prepared that hemodialysis may become necessary while awaiting a compatible match.

Concomitant or pretransplant nephrectomy is neither suggested nor commonly performed as the cystic kidneys are apt to reduce in size, thus negating the need to remove them.[18] There are a few special circumstances, however, in which there may be indications to remove the cystic kidneys before transplantation, which include a voluminous kidney that will not allow placement of the transplanted kidney, recurrent cystic hemorrhage or infection, nephrolithiasis with renal colic, and obstruction symptoms resulting from compression.[33]

The latter includes shortness of breath and gastrointestinal-related symptoms, such as nausea and vomiting and early satiety and retractable pain.

Below are valuable points in patient education:

- Disease course of ADPKD is variable even in those who have ADPKD1 variety
- Therapeutic lifestyle modifications are very important at a younger age than would normally be anticipated
- Some conditions may be more difficult to treat (e.g: osteoporosis as medications used to treat are nephrotoxic)
- Symptoms appear early in life particularly hypertension
- Lower blood pressure is desirable
- Other later symptoms include: abdominal distention, gross hematuria, early satiety, shortness of breath, constipation. These occur secondary to compression of structures by the enlarged cystic kidneys
- Pain is a common expected symptom and occurs due to different complications
- Cysts may rupture with trauma or spontaneously; therefore, it is important to avoid contact sports and other activities which may cause trauma resulting in cystic hemorrhage
- Once eGFR reaches 30 mL/min, decline may accelerate more rapidly
- Lifestyle and risk factor modifications can slow the progression of disease
- Cysts can develop in extrarenal locations, such as liver, pancreas, and so forth
- Many patients (but not all) progress to ESRD with best treatment being renal replacement with living donor transplant
- Quality of life can be improved by education, lifestyle modification, and renal replacement if indicated

NEPHROLOGY CONSULT

It is important that the primary care physician possess a high level of suspicion for patients who present with common symptoms, such as hypertension at a younger age, hematuria, and family history, because decline in renal function, as previously discussed, may not be evident although damage is occurring concurrently. Prompt diagnosis via ultrasound and referral to Nephrology is helpful for further delineation of severity of renal disease, determination of extrarenal complications, and extensive expectant management for patients and their families.

Initially after diagnosis, visits may occur every few years but, as CKD progresses, visits may likely be more frequent. The primary care physician and nephrologist work in concert to provide the optimal care for the patient until the time at which the nephrologist and transplant physicians coordinate care later in the disease.

SUMMARY

ADPKD is the most common inherited renal cystic disease that can result in ESRD necessitating renal transplant; however, its course, symptomology, and severity is often variable between patients. Although there are very limited targeted treatments at this time, risk factor reduction for renal failure as well as management of associated cardiovascular risk factors remains the essence of ADPKD treatment. There are disease-modifying treatments currently under investigation that may lead to discovery of methods of earlier intervention before irreversible renal damage. In the meantime, expedient diagnosis, lifestyle modifications, and extensive patient education are important modalities that are critical early on to reduce the burden associated with ADPKD and improve quality of life.

CLINICS CARE POINTS

- Early suspicion of ADPKD diagnosis is crucial to slow progression.
- Consider ADPKD in patients who have a family history and present with secondary hypertension, persistent flank pain or hematuria.
- Consider genetic counseling in conjunction with family planning and screening for potential family donors.
- Goals: Strict blood pressure control with a minimum goal of <130/80mm Hg; Restrict dietary sodium; Maintain BMI/weight in normal range; Follow guidelines for lipids based on CKD.
- Use imaging modalities to monitor disease progression as GRF is not correlative.
- Provide pain management for patients.
- Educate patients early on regarding disease progression and renal replacement.

ACKNOWLEDGMENTS

Thank you to Dr. Diane Beebe, Steve McDougald, Dr. Ashish Upadhyay and Dr. Anju Yadav for their support with this article.

DISCLOSURE

The authors have nothing to disclose.

REFERENCES

1. Beebe, D. Autosomal dominant polycystic kidney disease. Am Fam Physician. 96(53):925-930.

2. Kumar V, Abbas A, Aster J, et al. Robbins and Cotran pathologic basis of disease. Philadelphia: Elsevier Saunders; 2020.
3. Torra R. Recent advances in the clinical management of autosomal-dominant polycystic kidney disease. QJM 1996;89(11):803. www.ncbi.nim.nih.gov/pmc/articles. 2019 Jan 29.
4. Terryn S, Ho A, Beauwens R, et al. Fluid transport and cystogenesis in autosomal dominant polycystic kidney disease. Biochim Biophys Acta 2011;1812(10):1314–21.
5. Rahbari-Oskoui F, Williams O, Chapman A. Mechanisms and management of hypertension in autosomal dominant polycystic kidney disease. Nephrol Dial Transplant 2014;29(12):2194–201.
6. Cornec-Le Gall E, Alam A, Perrone RD. Autosomal dominant polycystic disease. Lancet 2019;393:919–35.
7. Helal I. Autosomal dominant polycystic kidney disease: new insights into treatment. Saudi J Kidney Dis Transpl 2013;24(2):230–4.
8. Hateboer N, v Dijk MA, Bogdanova N, et al. Comparison of phenotypes of polycystic kidney disease types 1 and 2. European PKD1-PKD2 Study Group. Lancet 1999;353:103–7.
9. Rangan G, Nankivell B. Management of autosomal dominant polycystic kidney disease. MedicineToday 2014;15(6):16–27.
10. Gimpel C, Bergmann C, Bockenhauer D, et al. International consensus statement on the diagnosis and management of autosomal dominant polycystic kidney disease in children and young people. Nat Rev Nephrol 2019;15:713–26.
11. Salvadori M, Tsalouchos A. New therapies targeting cystogenesis in autosomal polycystic kidney disease. EMJ Nephrol 2017;5(1):102–11.
12. Srivastava A, Patel N. Autosomal dominant polycystic kidney disease. Am Fam Physician 2014;90(5):303–7.
13. Torres JA, Rezaei M, Broderick C. Crystal deposition triggers tubule dilation that accelerates cystogenesis in polycystic kidney disease. J Clin Invest 2019;129(10):4506–22.
14. Agulari G, Catizone L, Del Senno L. Multidrug therapy for polycystic kidney disease: a review and perspective. Am J Nephrol 2013;37(2):175–82.
15. Torra R. Polycystic kidney disease clinical presentation. Medscape 2020;24. https://emedicine.medscape.com/article/244907-clinical.
16. Bello-Reuss E, Holubec K, Rajaraman S. Angiogenesis in autosomal-dominant polycystic kidney disease. Kidney Int 2001;60(1):37–45.
17. Chebib FT, Torres VE. Recent advances in the management of autosomal dominant polycystic kidney disease. Clin J Am Soc Nephrol 2016;13:1765–76.
18. Colbert GB, Elrggal ME, Gaur L, et al. Update and review of adult polycystic kidney disease. Dis Mon 2020;66(5):100887.
19. Ravine D, Gibson RN, Walker RG, et al. Evaluation of ultrasonographic diagnostic criteria for autosomal dominant polycystic kidney disease 1. Lancet 1994;343(8901):824.
20. Pei Y, Obaji J, Dupuis A, et al. Unified criteria for ultrasonographic diagnosis of ADPKD. J Am Soc Nephrol 2009;20(1):205–12.
21. Rastogi A, Ameen KM, Al-Baghdadi M, et al. Autosomal dominant polycystic kidney disease: updated perspectives. Ther Clin Risk Manag 2019;15:1041–52.
22. Cornec-LeGali E. The PROPKD score: a new algorithm to predict renal survival in autosomal polycystic kidney disease. J Am Soc Nephrol 2015;10:1681.
23. Wyatt C, Le Meur Y. REPRISE: tolvaptan in advanced polycystic kidney disease. Nephrology Digest Polycystic Kidney Disease 2018;93:292–5.

24. Chebib FT, Perrone RD, Chapman AB, et al. A practical guide for treatment of rapidly progressive ADPKD with tolvaptan. J Am Soc Nephrol 2018;29(10): 2458–70.
25. Schrier RW, Abebe KZ, Perrone RD, et al. Blood pressure in early autosomal dominant polycystic kidney disease. N Engl J Med 2014;371(24):2255–66.
26. Sallee M, Rafat C, Zahar J. Cyst Infections in Patients with Autosomal Dominant Polycystic Kidney Disease. Clin J Am Soc Nephrol 2009;4(7):1183–9.
27. Luciano RL, Dahl NK. Extra-renal manifestations of autosomal dominant polycystic kidney disease (ADPKD): considerations for routine screening and management. Nephrol Dial Transplant 2014;29(2):247–54.
28. Hughes PD, Becker GJ. Screening for intracranial aneurysms in autosomal dominant polycystic kidney disease. Nephrology (Carlton) 2003;8(4):163–70.
29. Bernts L, Drenth J, Tjwa E. Management of portal hypertension and ascites in polycystic liver disease. November 2019; Vol 39. Issue 11: 2024-2033.
30. Van Aaerts R, van de Laarschot L, Banales J. Clinical management of polycystic liver disease. J Hepatol 2018;68:827–37.
31. Spithoven EM, Kramer A, Meijer E, et al. Renal replacement therapy for autosomal dominant polycystic kidney disease (ADPKD) in Europe: prevalence and survival—an analysis of data from the ERA-EDTA Registry. Nephrol Dial Transplant 2014;29(Suppl 4):iv15.
32. Muller R-U, Benzing T. Management of autosomal-dominant polycystic kidney disease-state-of-the-art. Clin Kidney J 2018;11(suppl_1):i2–13.
33. Rastogi A, Mohammed A, Lerma E, et al. Autosomal dominant polycystic kidney disease: updated perspectives. Ther Clin Risk Manag 2019;15:1041–52.

Renal Repercussions of Medications

Rachel Shaddock, PharmD[a],*, Katherine Vogel Anderson, PharmD, BCACP[a],
Rebecca Beyth, MD[b]

KEYWORDS

- Drug-induced kidney injury • Geriatric medications • Acute kidney injury (AKI)
- Nephrotoxins

KEY POINTS

- Medications can cause acute injury to the kidneys, which can lead to collateral issues, such as chronic kidney disease (CKD), if the offending agent is not identified and discontinued in a timely manner.
- Some medications carry a higher risk of kidney injury than others, and prescriber awareness of such medications can help prevent increased mortality and morbidity associated with a drug-induced kidney injury.
- If nephrotoxic medications cannot be avoided, hydration, avoiding use with other nephrotoxic drugs, and using the lowest effective dose are strategies that can mitigate further damage.

INTRODUCTION

Medications can cause an acute injury to the kidneys that can lead to collateral issues, such as chronic kidney disease (CKD), if the offending agent is not identified and discontinued in a timely manner. Although there are multiple causes of renal injury, medications are a common cause of both acute kidney injury (AKI) and CKD. Nephrotoxic medications are responsible for 20% of hospitalizations for acute renal failure, and the mortality associated with AKI ranges from 23% to 80%, depending on if renal replacement therapy is required.[1,2] Awareness of these nephrotoxic agents when prescribing can help prevent the detrimental effects on the kidneys. Many medications are excreted by glomerular filtration or secretion into renal tubules, which, in turn, increases the potential for kidney injury.[3] This article highlights drug-induced kidney disease, renal repercussions of medications, and mechanisms of pharmacologic kidney injury.

[a] University of Florida College of Pharmacy, PO Box 100486, Gainesville, FL 32610-0486, USA;
[b] Division of Internal Medicine, University of Florida College of Medicine, NF/SG Veterans Health System GRECC, NF/SG VHS GRECC (182), 1601 Southwest Archer Road, Gainesville, FL 32608, USA
* Corresponding author.
E-mail address: rshaddock@cop.ufl.edu

Prim Care Clin Office Pract 47 (2020) 691–702
https://doi.org/10.1016/j.pop.2020.08.006   primarycare.theclinics.com

Based on data from prospective cohort studies of AKI, the incidence of drug-induced kidney disease ranges between 14% and 26%.[4] The incidence generally is higher in hospitalized patients, most often because of the use of contrast dyes for diagnostic testing while inpatient. Contrast dye can lead to the long-term complication called contrast-induced nephropathy, especially in the presence of concomitant nephrotoxic medications.

Drug-induced kidney injury also is prevalent in the outpatient setting and is especially concerning in the geriatric population because of polypharmacy. One cross-sectional analysis of Medicare claims data in 2016 found that 56.7% of elderly patients were on at least 5 prescription drugs, which is a dramatic increase from 39% in 2010.[5] Polypharmacy in the elderly is responsible for $1.3 billion in avoidable health care costs due to preventable hospitalizations and emergency room visits for adverse drug events, such as drug-induced kidney injury.[6]

Not only do geriatric patients take combinations of medications that have the potential to injure the kidneys but also age-based changes in pharmacokinetics; comorbidities, such as diabetes and heart failure; and preexisting renal impairment can increase the risk of kidney injury in geriatric patients.[7] Both glomerular filtration rate (GFR) and renal plasma flow declines with age, further escalating the geriatric population's risk of experiencing medication-related renal damage.[8] Medications that often are prescribed in the outpatient setting, which can lead to drug-induced kidney injury, are reviewed in the remainder of this article (**Table 1**).

ANTIMICROBIALS

Oral antimicrobials often are prescribed in the outpatient setting for cellulitis, sinusitis, and streptococcal pharyngitis. Although antimicrobials certainly are the standard of care for infectious disease management, they also can cause collateral damage because they are nephrotoxic.

Sulfamethoxazole/trimethoprim (Bactrim) is a common cause of drug-induced kidney injury. The mechanism of kidney injury is thought to be renal tubular necrosis and acute interstitial nephritis, leading to subsequent complications, such as hyperkalemia, crystalluria, and eventually renal failure.[9] Sulfa-containing medications, such as the sulfamethoxazole component of Bactrim, are excreted in large amounts in the urine. Because sulfa moieties are weak acids, they generally are insoluble in acidic urine. This leads to precipitation in the renal tubular lumen and, in turn, causes obstruction.[10]

In a retrospective study of 573 patients prescribed Bactrim, 11.2% developed AKI either during or immediately after a course of Bactrim therapy.[9] To rule out an acute infection as the cause of kidney injury, the comparator group included patients with similar demographics who were prescribed clindamycin rather than Bactrim. None of the patients in the comparator group experienced an AKI. The time to onset of kidney injury was as early as 3 days into treatment and as late as 2 days after completion of therapy. In the same trial, patients with uncontrolled diabetes were at a higher risk of developing kidney injury with the use of Bactrim.[9] Therefore, if clinically appropriate, it may be prudent to select an antimicrobial agent other than Bactrim for patients with poorly controlled diabetes, especially if treatment duration is expected to be greater than 3 days.

Fluoroquinolones also are associated with kidney injury. Although not as common as with sulfonamide-containing medications, ciprofloxacin (Cipro) and levofloxacin (Levaquin) can cause crystal-induced renal injury due to precipitation in the renal tubules and subsequent obstruction of urine output.[11] To avoid such renal

Table 1
Commonly used medications with potential nephrotoxicity

Medication	Mechanism of Renal Toxicity	Monitoring Strategies
Antimicrobials		
Sulfamethoxazole/ trimethoprim	Renal tubular necrosis and acute interstitial nephritis	Monitor serum creatinine and potassium when creatinine clearance <15 mL/min
Fluoroquinolones	Crystal nephropathy	No consensus for outpatient monitoring
Tenofovir	Acute tubular injury via mitochondrial toxin	When used for pre-exposure prophylaxis, monitor serum creatinine in 3 mo
NSAIDs	Causes vasoconstriction of afferent arteriole	No consensus for outpatient monitoring
Antihypertensive agents		
Diuretics (loop and thiazide)	AKI due to decreased renal perfusion	Monitor serum creatinine and electrolytes within 2 wk
ACE inhibitors/ARBs	Prevents angiotensin II's ability to constrict the efferent arteriole	Monitor serum creatinine and potassium within 2 wk
Statins	Development of rhabdomyolysis, leading to acute renal failure	Monitor creatine phosphokinase (CPK) and creatinine clearance when rhabdomyolysis symptoms present
Immunosuppressive agents		
Calcineurin inhibitors	Causes vasoconstriction of afferent and efferent arterioles	Monitor serum creatinine when using concomitant nephrotoxic agents
PPIs	Deposits in renal tubules causing acute interstitial nephritis	Monitor serum creatinine annually if long-term use

complications, it is important to limit fluoroquinolone use in patients with baseline renal impairment, adjust the dose of the fluoroquinolone according to creatinine clearance, and avoid fluoroquinolone use altogether in in patients who are volume depleted.

An antiretroviral agent known to cause kidney damage is tenofovir disoproxil fumarate (Viread). Tenofovir is a nucleotide reverse transcriptase inhibitor used in the treatment of human immunodeficiency virus and hepatitis B infections. Tenofovir is transported into the tubular cell cytoplasm via the human organic anion transporter, where it can cause injury if accumulation occurs.[12] Tenofovir is a mitochondrial toxin, which can lead to apoptosis and necrosis of the tubular cells, particularly in patients with genetic mutations in the efflux transporters responsible for removing tenofovir out of the tubular cells.[3] Subsequently, in the setting of reduced GFR, the transport of tenofovir into the tubular cells is increased, which further amplifies the risk of renal injury. To prevent renal injury associated with tenofovir, the general recommendation is to reduce the dose when creatinine clearance is calculated to be less than 50 mL/min[3]

A new prodrug formulation of tenofovir, known as tenofovir alafenamide (Vemlidy), results in lower plasma tenofovir concentrations than tenofovir disoproxil fumarate.[13] The risk of kidney injury is thought to increase with increased concentrations of tenofovir; therefore, the lower plasma concentrations associated with tenofovir alafenamide is associated with a lower incidence of kidney injury. A pooled analysis of 26 trials examining the rate of tenofovir discontinuation due to renal adverse events found a statistically significant reduction in discontinuation rates in the tenofovir alafenamide group (3/6360) compared with the tenofovir disoproxil fumarate group (14/2962).[13] Therefore, tenofovir alafenamide should be considered over tenofovir disoproxil fumarate, particularly in patients with preexisting kidney disease.

NONSTEROIDAL ANTI-INFLAMMATORY DRUGS

Nonsteroidal anti-inflammatory drugs (NSAIDs), such as ibuprofen (Motrin), naproxen (Aleve), and meloxicam (Mobic), adversely affect renal function. Prostaglandins in the kidneys are responsible for vasodilation of the renal vasculature.[14] Due to their inhibitory effects on prostaglandins, NSAIDs cause vasoconstriction of the afferent arteriole, thereby decreasing blood flow to the kidneys and increasing the risk of AKI and reduced renal function. The kidney injury associated with the use of NSAIDs is dose-dependent and the risk increases with duration of use. NSAID-induced kidney injury generally is reversible; however, a nested case-control study found that the risk of acute renal failure is 3-times higher in NSAID users compared with non-NSAID users.[15]

In addition to their direct effects on the kidneys via prostaglandin inhibition, NSAIDs can injure the kidneys indirectly by causing an increase in blood pressure. By increasing fluid and sodium retention, NSAIDs subsequently can increase blood pressure. As discussed previously, hypertension is a risk factor for AKI and CKD.[16] Therefore, caution should be used when prescribing NSAIDs in hypertensive patients regardless of kidney function. Ideally, patients with hypertension should avoid NSAIDs altogether to prevent renal impairment.

NSAIDs that are more selective for the cyclooxygenase-2 (COX-2) enzyme, known as COX-2 inhibitors, such as celecoxib (Celebrex), have a comparable risk of adverse effects on the kidneys. The COX-2 enzyme is expressed in the kidneys and, therefore, the effect of renal prostaglandin inhibition is similar.[17] Subsequently, celecoxib should be used cautiously in patients with impaired renal function, if not avoided altogether.

Of particular concern is that NSAIDs are available over the counter and often can be used by patients unbeknownst to the prescriber and the rest of the health care team. Therefore, it is important to assess over-the-counter drug use in all patients by taking a complete medication history and reconciling medication lists, especially in those who have reduced renal function or already are on other nephrotoxic medications. Strategies used to prevent drug-induced kidney injury from NSAIDs are to counsel the patient to use the shortest duration of therapy as possible, substitute for less nephrotoxic agents, such as acetaminophen (Tylenol), and to stay hydrated during NSAID therapy.[18] Additionally, prolonged NSAID therapy should be avoided in patients with GFR less than 60 mL/min and should be avoided altogether when GFR less than 30 mL/min.[19]

ANTIHYPERTENSIVE AGENTS

Adequately controlling blood pressure is imperative to prevent the progression of renal damage.[16] Attaining blood pressure control in hypertensive patients can be a daunting task because data suggest that more than 75% of patients with hypertension require more than 1 medication to achieve goal blood pressure.[20] Antihypertensive agents, however, also are associated with kidney injury. Diuretics are associated with an increased risk of kidney injury due to the pharmacologic action of volume depletion.

Angiotensin-converting enzyme (ACE) inhibitors and angiotensin II receptor blockers (ARBs) both have potential to cause renal dysfunction as well as the potential to preserve renal function via pharmacologic action on the kidneys.

Loop diuretics, including furosemide (Laxix), bumetanide (Bumex), and ethacrynic acid (Edecrin), and thiazide diuretics, including chlorthalidone (Thalitone), hydrochlorothiazide (Microzide), and indapamide (Lozol), are known to cause AKI. Diuretics work by manipulating renal excretion of both fluids and electrolytes to create an environment that promotes water loss to decrease blood pressure.[21] Loop diuretics work primarily in the ascending loop of Henle. Thiazide diuretics work in the cortical diluting segment of the ascending loop of Henle. Fluid loss decreases intravascular volume and leads to reductions in blood pressure. An adverse effect of such diuresis, however, is excessive intravascular depletion, which leads to decreased blood flow to the kidneys. Decreased blood flow to the kidneys results in vasoconstriction of the afferent arteriole, subsequently leading to prerenal injury. A risk factor for developing diuretic-associated kidney injury is a predisposition to reduced renal perfusion, as in the setting of renal artery stenosis and congestive heart failure.[22]

In practice, this prerenal injury most often is represented by an acute increase in serum creatinine and/or an increase in blood urea nitrogen, which often is reversible, either with discontinuation of the offending agent or with administration of fluids. Decreased renal perfusion also increases the likelihood of damage to the kidneys caused by concomitant nephrotoxic agents.[22] One method to decrease the risk of prerenal injury caused by diuretics is to monitor renal function and electrolytes within 2 weeks of initiating or changing the dose of a diuretic. A second method is to use the lowest effective diuretic dose. In a retrospective study of 131 cases of diuretic-associated kidney injury, it was determined that the risk of AKI was increased when using doses of Lasix greater than or equal to 120 mg per day.[22] Although 92.4% of the cases from this study involved loop diuretics, the same principle of using the lowest effective diuretic dose can be applied to thiazide diuretics as a strategy to prevent over-diuresis and subsequent diuretic-induced kidney injury.

The other class of antihypertensive agents that are associated with kidney injury acts on the renin-angiotensin system. ACE inhibitors and ARBs have both beneficial effects on the kidneys and potential to cause acute injury to the kidneys. Angiotensin II increases blood pressure by causing vasoconstriction. In the kidneys, angiotensin II is responsible for causing constriction of the efferent arteriole to increase GFR.[23] Because ACE inhibitors and ARBs inhibit angiotensin II, these medications prevent constriction of the efferent arteriole, which leads to a decrease in GFR. This acute change in GFR causes the kidney injury associated with ACE-inhibitors and ARBs. Hence, it is prudent to check serum creatinine and electrolytes within 2 weeks of initiation of an ACE inhibitor or an ARB to monitor renal function and assess for any potential acute injury.[23]

Data also show that ACE inhibitors and ARBs can prevent the progression of CKD. The Kidney Disease: Improving Global Outcomes 2012 chronic kidney disease guidelines recommend the use of an ACE inhibitor or ARB for diabetic patients with CKD and a urine albumin excretion ratio of 30 mg to 300 mg per 24 hours.[24] In nondiabetic patients, ACE inhibitors and ARBs are recommended when the urine albumin excretion ratio is greater than 300 mg per 24 hours.[24] Elevated urine albumin excretion ratios are indicative of CKD. ACE inhibitors and ARBs have been shown to decrease urine albumin levels, due to vasodilation and a decrease in GFR, as explained previously.

The Heart Outcomes Prevention Evaluation trial was a double-blind randomized controlled trial of patients with at least 1 cardiovascular disease risk factor[25]; 9297 patients without evidence of clinical proteinuria were randomized to receive either ramipril, 10 mg once daily, or placebo for mean follow-up period of 5 years.[25] The primary outcome of this study was a composite outcome of cardiovascular death, myocardial infarction, or stroke.[25] Secondary analyses were performed, however, looking specifically at albuminuria data.[26] It was determined that the use of ramipril prevented proteinuria as well as the development of microalbuminuria in both diabetic and nondiabetic patients by 13% compared with placebo.[26] Although both ACE inhibitors and ARBs can cause AKI, both also can provide renal protection. Therefore, it is prudent to monitor and tailor therapy to each patient.

STATINS

Statins, also known as HMG-CoA, reductase inhibitors, are used to lower lipids and to reduce the risk of cardiovascular disease. These medications do not affect kidney function or cause kidney injury in the traditional manner as most of the agents discussed thus far. Instead, statins have indirect effects on the kidneys, leading to the potential for kidney injury.[27] Atorvastatin (Lipitor), simvastatin (Zocor), rosuvastatin (Crestor), fluvastatin (Lescol), lovastatin (Mevacor), and pravastatin (Pravachol) have the potential to cause rhabdomyolysis. Rhabdomyolysis occurs after muscle injury, which leads to muscle fiber death and spilling of muscle components into the bloodstream.[28] Such muscle fiber components in the blood can damage the kidneys during glomerular filtration and excretion.[28] Risk factors for the development of rhabdomyolysis include age over 65 years, preexisting kidney dysfunction, higher doses of statins, and female gender.[29]

In order to prevent renal failure due to rhabdomyolysis, it is imperative to identify the symptoms to assist in earlier detection. Muscle weakness, decreased urine output, Coca-Cola–colored urine, and excessive fatigue are hallmark symptoms of rhabdomyolysis.[28] In addition, prescribers should be cognizant of drug interactions that can increase the concentration of statins and, therefore, increase the risk of rhabdomyolysis. Medications that inhibit cytochrome P 450 (CYP) 3A4 increase levels of simvastatin, atorvastatin, and lovastatin.[29] Grapefruit juice should be avoided with all statins. Concomitant use of gemfibrozil (Lopid), a fibric acid derivative, with a statin can increase the risk of developing rhabdomyolysis due to the additive risk of myopathy.[29] The combination of gemfibrozil with a statin should be avoided. If the combination is indicated, however, the lowest effective statin dose should be used and the patient should be monitored closely for symptoms of rhabdomyolysis.

IMMUNOSUPPRESSIVE AGENTS

Calcineurin inhibitors, such as tacrolimus (Prograf) and cyclosporine (Neoral), are associated with nephrotoxicity. These medications are used in transplant patients and to treat ulcerative colitis and rheumatoid arthritis. Calcineurin inhibitors cause immunosuppression by inhibiting T-cell activation through blocking calcineurin and interleukin 2. The incidence of nephrotoxicity with these medications has been well studied. In a cohort study of 69,321 nonrenal transplant patients from 1990 to 2000, the incidence of the development of CKD was 16.5% after a median follow-up period 3 years.[30] In a subset of 41,797 patients receiving cyclosporine had a 24% greater risk of developing chronic renal failure.[30] Therefore, this study proved that one of the risk factors for progression to CKD was the use of a calcineurin inhibitor.

Calcineurin is not specific to T cells. Inhibition of calcineurin in renal arterioles can lead to nephrotoxicity.[31] The mechanism by which calcineurin inhibitors cause nephrotoxicity is thought to be due to vasoconstriction of the afferent and efferent glomerular arterioles, which leads to decreased perfusion of the kidneys. Such vaso-constriction is hypothesized to be caused by a decrease in the production of vasodi-lators caused by the inhibition of calcineurin.[32] The risk of kidney injury increases with higher doses of calcineurin inhibitors. Other risk factors associated with calcineurin inhibitor-induced kidney injury include renal transplant, concomitant use of NSAIDs, diuretics, and medications that inhibit the metabolism of calcineurin inhibitors (eg, CYP inhibitors).[33]

Therapeutic drug monitoring (TDM) of calcineurin inhibitors is a useful strategy to prevent nephrotoxicity. To ensure efficacy and prevent toxicities, the 12-hour trough goal range for tacrolimus is 5 ng/mL to 15 ng/mL and for cyclosporine is 150 ng/mL to 300 ng/mL.[27] More narrow ranges are indicated based on the transplanted organ, the time from transplant date, and concomitant medications used.[27] Calcineurin inhib-itor levels should be drawn every other day immediately following the transplant until target levels are achieved and anytime there is a change in dose or change in renal function.[27] In addition, calcineurin inhibitors should not be used with medications that inhibit their metabolism, such as amiodarone, ketoconazole, and diltiazem. If the combination of these medications cannot be avoided, drug therapy monitoring should be tailored accordingly.[27] Some data suggests a benefit from using calcium channel blockers, such as diltiazem and nifedipine, to prevent the progression of cal-cineurin inhibitor nephrotoxicity. There is no evidence, however, to support that this increases graft survival.[34]

PROTON PUMP INHIBITORS

The proton pump inhibitors (PPIs), omeprazole (Prilosec), pantoprazole (Protonix), esomeprazole (Nexium), lansoprazole (Prevacid), dexlansoprazole (Dexilant), and rabeprazole (Aciphex), are prescribed for the treatment of gastroesophageal reflux disease and gastric and duodenal ulcers. Long-term use of PPIs is associated with acute interstitial nephritis. It is hypothesized that PPIs and their metabolites deposit into the interstitial space of the kidney tubules, leading to an immune response and subsequent kidney damage.[35] If left untreated, acute interstitial nephritis can lead to chronic interstitial nephritis and significantly increase the risk of developing CKD.[35]

The increased risk of AKI with the use of PPIs has been well studied. According to a population-based, nested, case-cohort study of 184,480 adult patients performed in the United States, the risk of AKI doubled in PPI users compared with the control pop-ulation.[36] Similarly, a Canadian study of 290,592 patients over the age of 65 revealed the risk of AKI was 2.5-times greater in those taking PPIs compared with those who are not. In addition, the same study also found the risk of acute interstitial nephritis, specifically, was 3-times higher in PPI users compared with the control group.[37] For patients with baseline renal disease, the risk of developing an AKI is 5-times higher in PPI users compared with non-PPI users.[38]

Like NSAIDs, PPIs are available over the counter. Therefore, PPI use should be considered a potential factor in every patient experiencing AKI with no apparent cause. To prevent acute interstitial nephritis with the use of PPIs, the lowest dose should be used. The risk of nephrotoxicity is greater with twice-daily dosing compared with once-daily dosing.[35] If a patient requires long-term use of a PPI, serum creatinine should be monitored annually.[39] If acid suppressive therapy is indicated, it may pru-dent to consider histamine-2 receptor antagonists, such as ranitidine (Zantac) and famotidine (Pepcid), in patients with renal impairment. Although histamine-2 receptor antagonists require dose adjustments based on renal function, the risk of AKI with these medications is lower compared with PPIs.

HERBAL SUPPLEMENTS

Dietary supplements and herbal products frequently are used by patients in the outpatient setting for the treatment of a variety of diagnoses, such as depression, hyperlipidemia, and several others. In fact, 75% of the American population reports to using an herbal supplement at some point in their lives.[40] Herbal supplements are not regulated by the Food and Drug Administration (FDA) in the same way as over-the-counter and prescription medications.[41] As such, it is difficult to accurately capture the incidence of adverse effects, such as nephrotoxicity, with herbal supplements due to the lack of postmarketing adverse event reporting that is required for drugs approved by the FDA.[41] Heavy metals and other undisclosed ingredients in herbal supplements have the potential to cause AKI.[41] Licorice, creatine phosphate, and caffeine are just a few natural products that have been associated with an increased risk of nephrotoxicity (**Box 1**).

Licorice (*Glycyrrhiza glabra*) is used for dry mouth, dyspepsia, and for the treatment of menopausal symptoms. Licorice has mineralocorticoid activity and can cause AKI by suppressing the renin-aldosterone system, leading to fluid retention and hypokalemia, which can exacerbate any preexisting kidney impairment.[41] For this reason, it is recommended to limit the duration of use to a maximum of 4 weeks to 6 weeks and to avoid use in any patient with impaired renal function. Furthermore, the mineralocorticoid activity of licorice can worsen hypertension thereby indirectly damaging the kidneys.[41]

Creatine phosphate is an herbal supplement used most commonly to increase muscle strength and performance. Creatine phosphate in skeletal muscles serves as a precursor to phosphate, which is needed to regenerate adenosine triphosphate to improve muscle performance during exercise.[29] There have been few studies examining the nephrotoxicity of creatine; however, there have been several case reports highlighting renal insufficiency in young men taking creatine phosphate at doses ranging from 10 g to 20 g daily.[42,43] The renal impairment seen in these patients was reversed when creatine phosphate was discontinued.[42,43]

Caffeine is used for the treatment of headaches, weight loss, memory, and attention-deficit/hyperactivity disorder. In addition, caffeine is found as an adjuvant in combination pain products. Caffeine has been associated with an increased risk of calcium oxalate kidney stone formation.[44] Such risk was seen when caffeine was used at doses between 1 g and 4.8 g per day. In addition to stone formation, caffeine has a diuretic-like effect, which can lead to intravascular depletion and, therefore, decreased perfusion to the kidneys.[45]

STRATEGIES TO PREVENT DRUG-INDUCED NEPHROTOXICITY

There are several strategies practitioners can employ to prevent drug-induced nephrotoxicity, some of which have been discussed throughout this article (**Box 2**). First, it is prudent to avoid concomitant use of nephrotoxic medications, especially in patients who already are at risk for renal dysfunction. For example, the combination of tenofovir

---

Box 1
Herbal supplements

Licorice	Sodium and water retention and renin-aldosterone suppression
Creatine phosphate	Acute interstitial nephritis
Caffeine	Increased risk of kidney stone formation

Box 2
Strategies to prevent drug-induced kidney injury

- Avoid concomitant use of nephrotoxic agents.
- Ensure adequate hydration to ensure renal perfusion.
- Utilize therapeutic drug monitoring for efficacy and toxicity.
- Use lowest effective dose of nephrotoxic agents.
- Use the shortest duration of therapy to prevent injury to the kidneys.
- Monitor kidney function and consider dose reduction/discontinuation of injury occurs.

---

and NSAIDs can cause acute renal failure requiring hospitalization as well as renal replacement therapy. Although both medications individually increase the risk of drug-induced kidney injury, when used together, the risk is increased further. Therefore, avoiding the combination of nephrotoxic agents, when possible, can prevent additive adverse effects.

Another strategy to prevent renal damage is to ensure adequate hydration. This recommendation can be used for any patient; however, caution should be used in patients with heart failure who are at risk for fluid overload. Adequate hydration is defined as 3.7 L of water for men and 2.7 L for women.[46] Ample hydration helps increase intravascular volume to ensure renal perfusion and can help prevent kidney injury especially in the presence of nephrotoxic medications.

TDM is a third strategy used to prevent drug toxicity in patients with renal impairment.[47] Although TDM is used more frequently in the inpatient setting, there is a place in therapy for TDM in the outpatient setting as well. For example, the calcineurin inhibitors are monitored via TDM in an attempt to prevent nephrotoxicity, which is more likely to occur when drug concentrations are elevated.[26] In addition, warfarin is a common medication whose levels are monitored frequently to ensure efficacy and prevent toxicity.[47] In the setting of renal impairment, TDM is beneficial, given the variability of pharmacokinetic properties that can be impacted. Considerations, such as route of administration, timing of the last dose, and amount of the medication given, must be examined in order to properly interpret TDM levels.[47]

Lastly, if nephrotoxic agents cannot be avoided altogether, using the lowest effective dose and the shortest duration of therapy can prevent injury to the kidneys. It is reasonable to monitor renal function during the course of therapy with nephrotoxic medications to identify an acute injury before a chronic issue or complication arises. If there is an apparent injury to the kidneys either through an elevated serum creatinine or an elevated blood urea nitrogen level, it may be appropriate to discontinue the offending agent or reduce the dose, depending on the clinical picture and necessity of the medication.

SUMMARY

Primary care physicians often manage a majority of a patient's chronic conditions; therefore, it is imperative to be vigilant in maintaining a high index of suspicion for the potential of renal injury when prescribing medications.

The kidneys play a vital role in medication excretion. In addition, impaired kidney function can decrease drug elimination leading to an increased risk of side effects of certain medications. For these reasons, renal function is a patient-specific factor that always should be considered when selecting medications.

Furthermore, there are several classes of medications that can be directly toxic to the kidneys. Antimicrobials, NSAIDs, and antihypertensive agents can alter renal physiology. In patients with preexisting kidney disease, nephrotoxic medications should be avoided as much as possible. If nephrotoxic medications cannot be avoided, hydration, avoiding use with other nephrotoxic drugs, and using the lowest effective dose are strategies that can mitigate further damage.

When prescribing medications, the risks of adverse effects and the pharmacologic benefits of the medication always must be considered in an attempt to circumvent avoidable harm to the patient. As highlighted in this article, some medications carry a higher risk of kidney injury than others, and prescriber awareness of such medications can help prevent increased mortality and morbidity associated with a drug-induced kidney injury.

DISCLOSURE

The authors have nothing to disclose.

REFERENCES

1. Nolin TD, Himmelfarb J, Matzke GR. Drug-induced kidney disease. In: Pharmacotherapy. 6th edition. New York: McGraw-Hill; 2005. p. 871–87.
2. Uchino S. The epidemiology of acute renal failure in the world. Curr Opin Crit Care 2006;12:538–43.
3. Perazella MA. Drug-induced acute kidney injury: diverse mechanisms of tubular injury. Curr Opin Crit Care 2019;25(6):550–7.
4. Perazella MA. Pharmacology behind common drug nephrotoxicities. Clin J Am Soc Nephrol 2018;13(12):1897–908.
5. Ellenbogen MI, Wang P, Overton HN, et al. Frequency and predictors of polypharmacy in us medicare patients: a cross-sectional analysis at the patient and physician levels. Drugs & aging 2019;29:1–9.
6. Aitken M, Valkova S. Avoidable costs in US healthcare: the $200 billion opportunity from using medicines more responsibly. IMS Institute for Healthcare Informatics 2013;27–9.
7. Naughton CA. Drug-induced nephrotoxicity. Am Fam Physician 2008;78(6): 743–50.
8. Hämmerlein A, Derendorf H, Lowenthal DT. Pharmacokinetic and pharmacodynamic changes in the elderly. Clin Pharm 1998;35(1):49–64.
9. Fraser TN, Avellaneda AA, Graviss EA, et al. Acute kidney injury associated with trimethoprim/sulfamethoxazole. J Antimicrob Chemother 2012;67(5):1271–7.
10. Perazella MA. Crystal-induced acute renal failure. Am J Med 1999;106(4): 459–65.
11. Shahrbaf FG, Assadi F. Drug-induced renal disorders. J Renal Inj Prev 2015; 4(3):57.
12. Jafari A, Khalili H, Dashti-Khavidaki S. Tenofovir-induced nephrotoxicity: incidence, mechanism, risk factors, prognosis and proposed agents for prevention. Eur J Clin Pharmacol 2014;70(9):1029–40.
13. Gupta SK, Post FA, Arribas JR, et al. Renal safety of tenofovir alafenamide vs. tenofovir disoproxil fumarate: a pooled analysis of 26 clinical trials. AIDS 2019; 33(9):1455.
14. Blowey DL. Nephrotoxicity of over-the-counter analgesics, natural medicines, and illicit drugs. Adolesc Med Clin 2005;16(1):31–43.

15. Huerta C, Castellsague J, Varas-Lorenzo C, et al. Nonsteroidal anti-inflammatory drugs and risk of ARF in the general population. Am J Kidney Dis 2005;45:531–9.
16. Centers for Disease Control and Prevention. Chronic kidney disease in the United States, 2019. Atlanta (GA): US Department of Health and Human Services, Centers for Disease Control and Prevention; 2019.
17. Harris RC. COX-2 and the kidney. J Cardiovasc Pharmacol 2006;47:S37–42.
18. Munar MY, Singh H. Drug dosing adjustments in patients with chronic kidney disease. Am Fam Physician 2007;75(10):1487–96.
19. Levin A, Stevens PE, Bilous RW, et al. KDIGO 2012 clinical practice guideline for the evaluation and management of chronic kidney disease. Kidney Int Suppl 2013;3(1):1–50.
20. Gradman AH, Basile JN, Carter BL, et al, American Society of Hypertension Writing Group. Combination therapy in hypertension. J Am Soc Hypertens 2010;4(2):90–8.
21. Rose BD. Diuretics. Kidney Int 1991;39:336.
22. Wu X, et al. Diuretics associated acute kidney injury: clinical and pathological analysis. Ren Fail 2014;36(7):1051–5.
23. Navis G, Faber HJ, de Zeeuw D, et al. ACE inhibitors and the kidney. Drug Saf 1996;15(3):200–11.
24. Kidney Disease: Improving Global Outcomes (KDIGO) Blood Pressure Work Group. KDIGO Clinical Practice Guideline for the Management of Blood Pressure in Chronic Kidney Disease. Kidney inter, Suppl 2012;2:337–414.
25. Yusuf S, Sleight P, Pogue JF, et al. Effects of an angiotensin-converting-enzyme inhibitor, ramipril, on cardiovascular events in high-risk patients. N Engl J Med 2000;342(3):145–53.
26. Mann JF, Gerstein HC, Yi QL, et al. Development of renal disease in people at high cardiovascular risk: results of the HOPE randomized study. J Am Soc Nephrol 2003;14:641–7.
27. Kidney Disease: Improving Global Outcomes (KDIGO) Transplant Work Group. KDIGO clinical practice guideline for the care of kidney transplant recipients. Am J Transplant 2009;9:S1.
28. Petejova N, Martinek A. Acute kidney injury due to rhabdomyolysis and renal replacement therapy: a critical review. Crit Care 2014;18(3):224.
29. Schech S, Graham D, Staffa J, et al. Risk factors for statin-associated rhabdomyolysis. Pharmacoepidemiol Drug Saf 2007;16(3):352–8.
30. Ojo AO, Held PJ, Port FK, et al. Chronic renal failure after transplantation of a non-renal organ. N Engl J Med 2003;349(10):931–40.
31. Liu EH, Siegel RM, Harlan DM, et al. T cell-directed therapies: lessons learned and future prospects. Nat Immunol 2007;8:25–30.
32. Lanese DM, Conger JD. Effects of endothelin receptor antagonist on cyclosporine-induced vasoconstriction in isolated rat renal arterioles. J Clin Invest 1993;91(5):2144–9.
33. Naesens M, Kuypers DR, Sarwal M. Calcineurin inhibitor nephrotoxicity. Clin J Am Soc Nephrol 2009;4(2):481–508.
34. Chrysostomou AN, Walker RG, Russ GR, et al. Diltiazem in renal allograft recipients receiving cyclosporine. Transplantation 1993;55(2):300–4.
35. Eusebi LH, Rabitti S, Artesiani ML, et al. "proton pump inhibitors: risks of long-term use.". J Gastroenterol Hepatol 2017;32(7):1295–302.
36. Klepser DG, Collier DS, Cochran GL. Proton pump inhibitors and acute kidney injury: a nested case–control study. BMC Nephrol 2013;14:150.

37. Antoniou T, Macdonald EM, Hollands S, et al. Proton pump inhibitors and the risk of acute kidney injury in older patients: a population-based cohort study. CMAJ Open 2015;3:E166–71.
38. Blank ML, Parkin L, Paul C, et al. A nationwide nested case–control study indicates an increased risk of acute interstitial nephritis with proton pump inhibitor use. Kidney Int 2014;86:837–44.
39. International Society of Nephrology. Summary of recommendation statements. Kidney Int Suppl 2013;3:5–14.
40. Barrett B, Kiefer D, Rabago D. Assessing the risks and benefits of herbal medicine: an overview of scientific evidence. Altern Ther Health Med 1999;5(4):40.
41. Bagnis CI, Deray G, Baumelou A, et al. Herbs and the kidney. Am J kidney Dis 2004;44(1):1.
42. Koshy KM, Griswold E, Schneeberger EE. Interstitial nephritis in a patient taking creatine. N Engl J Med 1999;340:814–5.
43. Kuehl K, Goldberg L, Elliot D. Renal insufficiency after creatine supplementation in a college football athlete. Med Sci Sports Exerc 1998;30(5 Suppl):S235.
44. Massey LK, Sutton RA. Acute caffeine effects on urine composition and calcium kidney stone risk in calcium stone formers. J Urol 2004;172(2):555–8.
45. Peerapen P, Thongboonkerd V. Caffeine in kidney stone disease: risk or benefit? Adv Nutr 2018;9(4):419–24.
46. Campbell S. Dietary reference intakes: water, potassium, sodium, chloride, and sulfate. Clinical Nutrition Insight 2004;30(6):1–4.
47. Witt DM, Holbrook A, Schulman S, et al. Evidence-based management of anticoagulant therapy. Chest 2012;141(2):e152S–84S.

Care of the Renal Transplant Patient

Jennifer G. Foster, MD, MBA[a],*, Keith J. Foster, MD, MBA[b]

KEYWORDS

- Renal transplant ● Kidney transplant ● Transplantation ● End stage renal disease

KEY POINTS

- Candidates for renal transplant undergo an extensive preoperative evaluation in order to optimize their medical condition for surgery.
- Renal transplant patients typically receive induction and then maintenance immunosuppression to maintain a functioning allograft.
- Rejection of the allograft requires high clinical suspicion in order to initiate or augment current treatment to preserve the graft.
- Renal transplant patients require ongoing surveillance and monitoring in the primary care setting for common issues like osteoporosis, cardiovascular disease, and malignancy.

INTRODUCTION

Renal transplantation is the treatment of choice for advanced chronic kidney disease (CKD) and has been shown to afford patients a better quality of life compared with dialysis.[1] After years of a widening gap between organ supply and patients receiving transplants in the United States, in recent years, the number of both deceased and living donor renal transplant surgeries performed in the United States has been increasing, and the number of patients waiting for a kidney transplant has started to decrease, somewhat narrowing this gap. The number of patients nationally maintaining a functioning renal allograft is forecast to be more than 250,000 in the next 1 to 2 years.[2] As a result, primary care providers need to be well equipped to care for renal transplant patients now more than ever.

INDICATIONS AND CONTRAINDICATIONS TO RENAL TRANSPLANTATION

The indication for renal transplant is advanced, irreversible CKD. Patients should be referred to a transplant center when their glomerular filtration rate falls below

[a] Charles E. Schmidt College of Medicine, Florida Atlantic University, 777 Glades Road, ME-104, Boca Raton, FL 33431, USA; [b] Broward Health North, 201 East Sample Road, Deerfield Beach, FL 33064, USA
* Corresponding author.
E-mail address: fosterj@health.fau.edu

Prim Care Clin Office Pract 47 (2020) 703–712
https://doi.org/10.1016/j.pop.2020.08.007
0095-4543/20/Published by Elsevier Inc.
primarycare.theclinics.com

30 mL/min/1.73 m². ³ This allows for ample time for the patient to undergo an appropriate recipient evaluation (described later) and explore options for a donor kidney.

Absolute contraindications to renal transplantation include:

- Active infection
- Active malignancy
- Ongoing substance abuse
- Uncontrolled psychiatric disease
- Documented ongoing nonadherence to medical therapy
- A decreased life expectancy

In general, most transplant centers deem candidates with a life expectancy less than 1 year ineligible for surgery. The current standard of care is to transplant candidates for both living and deceased renal grafts with a life expectancy of at least 5 years, due to the documented benefit of renal transplantation over dialysis only after the initial perioperative period.[4] Due to the need for immunosuppressive medications after the transplant, most centers do not transplant patients with overt acquired immunodeficiency syndrome and active hepatitis B, because the further immunosuppression with medications postoperatively would further increase the risk for opportunistic infection. In addition, patients with disseminated or untreated malignancy or severe degrees of comorbid conditions (ie, irreparable coronary artery disease) either have a lower life expectancy or often are poor surgical candidates and deemed ineligible for renal transplantation. Immunologic contraindications include the presence of antibodies against the ABO blood group antigens or against the HLA, because these potentially cause hyperacute rejection in the immediate postoperative period.[4]

Relative contraindications to renal transplantation sometimes are uncovered during the recipient evaluation, including moderately severe degrees of comorbid conditions (ie, chronic liver disease and structural heart disease), severe hyperparathyroidism, and systemic diseases causing renal failure (ie, systemic lupus erythematosus). Some centers are cautious in transplanting patients who have primary renal diseases like multiple myeloma or amyloidosis due to the high mortality rate of these diseases.[5] Infection with human immunodeficiency virus (HIV) or hepatitis C previously was an absolute contraindication to transplantation; however, with the advent of better antiretroviral therapy for HIV and direct antiviral medications for hepatitis C, more and more centers are performing renal transplants for patients with these diseases.[4]

EVALUATION OF CANDIDATES FOR TRANSPLANT

A potential recipient for a renal transplant undergoes an extensive immunologic and infectious work-up, in addition to further testing for malignancy and comorbid conditions as dictated by a patient's entire medical history and physical examination. Immunologic testing includes ABO blood group and HLA typing, as discussed previously. HLA typing matches the recipient with potential donors. The evaluation for infectious disease, includes serologic testing for varicella, rubella, measles, and mumps viruses. If a potential recipient is found to be nonimmune to these diseases, it is recommended that they become vaccinated prior to transplantation. Other tests include those for cytomegalovirus (CMV), Epstein-Barr virus (EBV), HIV, hepatitis B and hepatitis C, tuberculosis, and syphilis.[4]

Additionally, a potential recipient receives other tests based on age, gender, and comorbidities. Routine preoperative testing includes chest radiography and electrocardiogram, but the presence of cardiac risk factors may prompt additional cardiovascular testing. Imaging also often is performed on the renal anatomy and genitourinary tract with ultrasound as well. Candidates also must undergo all age-appropriate and gender-appropriate cancer screenings prior to transplantation, including Pap smear, colonoscopy, and mammogram. Baseline bone mineral density screening often is performed with dual energy x-ray absorptiometry (DXA) prior to transplant, because renal transplant recipients are at a high risk for bone disease long term. Finally, all candidates for renal transplantation also undergo psychosocial evaluation, to assess for any barriers to adherence to the perioperative and postoperative treatment plan, especially those barriers to the need for lifelong immunosuppressive therapy.[6] Patient education on diet and nutrition, activity, and complications of transplant varies depending on the transplant center, however, the US Department of Agriculture and Food and Drug Administration has written a guide for solid organ transplant recipients, which provides patients with important information regarding food safety so as to avoid food-borne illnesses, which ultimately can be lengthier and more severe in post-transplant patients, resulting in hospitalization and even death. The main recommendation includes avoidance of undercooked or raw meat, fish, and eggs.

Patients are also typically required to obtain a dental examination prior to transplant and should not have elective dental work for the first 6 months post-transplant, due to the risk for infection.

KEY CONCEPTS OF RENAL TRANSPLANT SURGERY

Transplanted kidneys originate from both living and deceased donors. Once the allograft is procured from the donor, it is preserved and cooled before being implanted into the recipient. Because of its proximity to the bladder and iliac vessels, the iliac fossa typically is the ideal location for the allograft. In addition, a donor's renal vessels are usually transplanted with the kidney and attached to the receipient's iliac vessels in an end-to-side fashion, minimizing the stenosis that can later occur with an end-to-end anastomosis.[7] A few different approaches exist to establish urinary drainage, depending on the donor's ureter length and recipient's history of bladder issues or prior surgical procedures.

Living-donor allografts have a longer short-term survival than similarly matched deceased-donor allografts.[8] This reflects the suboptimal tissue conditions of the deceased-donor allografts due to ischemia as well as the potential for reperfusion injury. This trend in improved survival extends out to both 5 years and 10 years post-transplant as well.[4]

IMMUNOSUPPRESSION

Immunosuppression after a renal transplant occurs in 2 phases: induction and maintenance. The induction phase begins immediately postoperatively, often consisting of antibody-based therapy that aims to prevent acute rejection of the graft. The maintenance phase begins a few days postoperatively and continues for the life of the transplant. In this initial postoperative period, when immunosuppression is at its highest, renal transplant patients also receive prophylaxis against a variety of opportunistic infections. Trimethoprim/sulfamethoxazole is used to protect against *Pneumocystis jirovecii* pneumonia (PJP) and toxoplasmosis for the first 6 months to 1 year post-transplant.[9] Valganciclovir is used to prevent CMV reactivation in CMV-seropositive recipients and recipients with CMV-seropositive donors in the first 3 months to 1 year post-transplant[10] as well.

Maintenance immunosuppression consists of a combination of medications of different mechanisms of action that vary by patient and transplant center. Initial maintenance regimens often include a calcineurin inhibitor (CNI), an antimetabolite, and a glucocorticoid.[11] The most commonly used immunosuppressive medications are reviewed, because primary care providers should be aware of their side effects and potential long-term adverse effects as well (Table 1).

Calcineurin Inhibitors

CNIs work by blocking the production of interleukin 2, thereby inhibiting T-cell proliferation.[7] Cyclosporine and tacrolimus are the CNIs used most commonly, and 1 of these 2 medications is used in greater than 90% of all renal transplants in the United States.[12] Side effects of these medications include tremor, diabetes, hepatotoxicity, and, ironically, nephrotoxicity. Tacrolimus is more popular because it is associated with decreased rejection rates and is of similar cost. Tacrolimus also does not frequently cause hypertrichosis or gingival hyperplasia, as cyclosporine does. Because most drug interactions with CNIs are related to the hepatic cytochrome P450 system, transplant recipients on these medications should not eat grapefruit or drink grapefruit juice.[13]

Purine Antimetabolites

Medications in the purine antimetabolite class include azathioprine and mycophenolate mofetil (MMF). These medications inhibit purine synthesis and, therefore, inhibit the proliferation of both B cells and T cells, but they each do so in a slightly different pathway. The metabolites of azathioprine are incorporated into DNA and/or RNA transcription, halting the process altogether.[7] Side effects of azathioprine include bone marrow suppression (leukopenia to a greater degree than thrombocytopenia or anemia), jaundice, alopecia, and increased risk for neoplasia. The leukopenia caused often requires an adjustment in dose.

Alternatively, MMF inhibits an enzyme that is crucial for de novo purine synthesis, inosine monophosphate dehydrogenase. It causes less bone marrow suppression; however, other side effects include gastrointestinal upset and pure red cell aplasia.[7] Although azathioprine was an incredibly important medication during the advent of renal transplantation and is cheaper in cost, MMF has demonstrated a greater ability to prevent acute rejection and a cleaner side-effect profile, so it is now used more widely, in greater than 90% of transplants.[12]

Table 1
Immunosuppressive medications used in renal transplant

Medication	Class	Nonrenal Side Effects
Cyclosporine	CNI	Hypertrichosis, gingival hyperplasia, gynecomastia, hyperuricemia, gout, hyperlipidemia
Tacrolimus	CNI	Alopecia, post-transplantation diabetes
Azathioprine	Purine antimetabolite	Bone marrow suppression, hepatitis, cholestasis
MMF	Purine antimetabolite	Heartburn, nausea, diarrhea
Prednisone	Glucocorticoid	Osteoporosis, impaired wound healing, hyperlipidemia, glucose intolerance, psychiatric effects
Sirolimus Everolimus	mTOR inhibitor mTOR inhibitor	Impaired wound healing, reduced testosterone concentration, painful mouth ulcers, hyperlipidemia, thrombocytopenia, diarrhea, hyperlipidemia

Glucocorticoids

Glucocorticoids inhibit the transcription of numerous inflammatory cytokines and are a well-known adjunctive medication for renal transplant patients. They also have fairly notorious side effects, including osteopenia/osteoporosis; increased risk for infection, peptic ulcers, myopathy, cataracts, hypertension, and hyperglycemia; as well as the characteristic physical effects of moon facies, truncal obesity, striae, and cervicodorsal fat redistribution.[14] Higher doses of intravenous steroid are given intraoperatively during renal transplant. The medication then is switched to the oral formulation and the dose is tapered slowly. Many centers now have protocols for steroid avoidance or discontinuance due to the well-known adverse effects of these medications.[4] Primary care providers must be aware of and vigilant in monitoring the side effects of glucocorticoids.

Mammalian Target of Rapamycin Inhibitors

Mammalian target of rapamycin (mTOR) inhibitors include the medications sirolimus and everolimus. Their mechanism of action is the inhibition of T-cell growth factor pathways, preventing a systemic response to inflammatory cytokines.[4] When used, sirolimus often is administered along with MMF as a CNI-sparing agent, particularly in cases of CNI nephrotoxicity or other severe, persistent side effects from CNIs.[15] Side effects of sirolimus include hyperlipidemia, thrombocytopenia, and oral ulcers. Everolimus has a similar side-effect profile but better bioavailability compared with sirolimus.

GRAFT REJECTION

Graft rejection is mediated by both T cells and/or antibodies, causing a deterioration in renal function associated with specific histologic changes seen on biopsy of the graft. Rejection is classified based on pathogenesis and time of onset into 3 main types: hyperacute, acute, and chronic.[7] Hyperacute rejection occurs within minutes to hours post-transplant, when antibodies bind to the vasculature of the graft. The result is a grossly mottled-appearing, cyanotic organ that demonstrates areas of ischemic necrosis on graft biopsy. Thankfully, blood typing and cross-matching as well as the testing for HLAs have minimized such immunogenic incompatibility, thereby making the incidence of hyperacute rejection very rare.

Acute rejection is the most common form of rejection, occurring days to months post-transplant. Most patients are asymptomatic, presenting only with an increase in creatinine or proteinuria. Occasionally, patients present with fever, oliguria, and pain or tenderness to palpation of the graft.[4] Diagnosis is confirmed with biopsy of the graft demonstrating a lymphocytic infiltration in the tubules and interstitium. Biopsy also can determine the extent of the injury to the graft. Treatment of acute rejection is with increased immunosuppressive medications.

Chronic rejection, also called chronic renal allograft nephropathy, occurs over the course of several years, presenting at least 1 year after transplant.[7] The pathogenesis is poorly understood, and there are no standardized criteria by which to diagnose chronic rejection. Patients present with gradually worsening plasma creatinine levels, proteinuria, and/or hypertension. Biopsy of the graft can demonstrate pathology to all aspects of the renal parenchyma, including the vasculature, glomeruli, and tubules. Management of chronic rejection is individualized to each patient but typically includes the augmentation of their maintenance immunosuppressive regimen as well as the addition of an angiotensin-converting enzyme inhibitors or angiotensin receptor blockers.[16]

PRIMARY CARE ISSUES IN RENAL TRANSPLANT PATIENTS

Renal transplant patients are at risk for multiple issues and complications even after a successful transplant and with a functioning allograft, due to both the side effects from their immunosuppressive medications and the comorbidities that caused or came about as a result of their underlying chronic renal failure. These complications can be life threatening or threaten the life of the graft if not suspected and treated appropriately.

Infectious Diseases

Renal transplant patients are at risk for infectious complications, both common and opportunistic infections, due to the immunosuppression required post-transplant (**Table 2**). These infections can vary based on the time after surgery and degree of overall immunosuppression but are most common in the first 3 months post-transplant due to induction immunosuppressive therapy.[17]

In the immediate 1 month after transplant surgery, the most common infections are related to those derived from the donor or to the surgery itself. Donor-derived infections with multidrug-resistant bacteria are becoming more prevalent, despite surgical antibiotic prophylaxis, as the prevalence of these infections rises in general.[18] Infections that were present previously in the donor can also reemerge after transplant, including hepatitis B, hepatitis C, and tuberculosis, which illustrates the importance of a thorough infectious disease work-up prior to organ donation. Infections related to the surgery itself can include urinary tract infections (UTIs), central line–associated bloodstream infections (CLABSIs), and surgical site infections.

Infections in the first 1 month to 6 months post-transplant reflect the effect of maximal immunosuppression and, therefore, include many of the opportunistic infections. These include PJP, viral infections like CMV and EBV, geographically related fungal infections like histoplasmosis or blastomycosis, and tuberculosis and nontuberculous mycobacteria.[19] It is important to have a high suspicion for such infections in order to employ an appropriate diagnostic workup and antibiotic treatment. After the 6-month mark, patients still can be susceptible to these infections, with the

Table 2 Common infections in posttransplant period		
Early (<1 mo After Transplant)	**1–6 mo After Transplant**	**Late (>6 mo After Transplant)**
Staphylococcus aureus	CMV	CMV
Gram-negatives	EBV (including PTLD)	EBV (including PTLD)
Clostridium difficile	HSV	
Candida	VZV	VZV
Aspergillus	Polyoma (BK virus) PJP	Polyoma (BK virus)
Surgical site infections	*Toxoplasma gondii*	*Listeria*
Nosocomial PNA	*Listeria*	CAPs
CLABSIs	*Legionella*	*Nocardia*
UTIs	*Nocardia*	UTIs
TB reactivation Hepatitis B and C	Fungal infections TB reactivation Hepatitis B and C	

Abbreviations: CAP, community acquired pneumonia; HSV, herpes simplex virus; PNA, pneumonia; PTLD, post-transplant lymphoproliferative disorder, TB, uberculosis; VZV, varicella zoster virus.

addition of organisms like *Listeria*, *Nocardia*, and viruses more specific to renal transplant like the BK and JC polyomaviruses. BK virus is especially important to suspect and diagnose appropriately, because the clinical presentation can mimic that of acute rejection. Because the treatment of BK virus is a reduction of immunosuppression, whereas the treatment of acute rejection is an increase in immunosuppression, it is essential to delineate the cause of a patient's presentation to ensure appropriate treatment and preserved functioning of the allograft.[20]

Osteoporosis

Several risk factors contribute to bone loss in renal transplant patients, including pre-existing renal osteodystrophy and persistent hyperparathyroidism caused by the underlying chronic renal failure as well as glucocorticoid and CNI use post-transplant. As discussed previously, candidates for renal transplant often undergo screening DXA as part of the initial preoperative evaluation. Although the optimal interval between DXA testing in renal transplant patients is unknown, those patients at the highest risk of fracture include those with prior fracture, history of osteoporosis pretransplant, or history of osteopenia with either another risk factor for fracture or whose immunosuppression regimen is anticipated to include corticosteroids.[21] These high-risk patients should be monitored yearly or every other year with DXA testing. In addition to lifestyle changes and calcium and vitamin D replacement, persistent hyperparathyroidism should be treated, and the lowest dose of corticosteroid should be used for immunosuppression. The optimal treatment of osteoporosis in renal transplant patients is unknown; the typical approach is similar to that used in patients with CKD, beginning with bisphosphonates and reserving denosumab for patients who cannot take bisphosphonates.

Hematologic Issues

Renal transplant patients are susceptible to bone marrow suppression due largely in part to side effects from their immunosuppressive medications. These issues include leukopenia (either neutropenia, lymphocytopenia, or both), anemia, or thrombocytopenia. The patient's transplant nephrologist often adjusts the dosage of the medication thought to be causing leukopenia or thrombocytopenia.

Anemia is treated in a thoughtful and cautious manner. Although there is no target hemoglobin level in renal transplant patients, the use of iron, whether intravenous or oral, is safe and efficacious in restoring iron stores post-transplant. Erythropoietin-stimulating agents (ESAs) also have been studied in the renal transplant population and do not confer any improvement in hemoglobin in the first 3 months post-transplant; additionally, ESAs have the potential for thrombotic effects, so they are not recommended in this initial postoperative period.[22] Clinicians must also remember that gastrointestinal bleeding is a potential side effect from high-dose and long-term steroid use and should be ruled out in this population. Transfusions generally are avoided post-transplant in order to prevent alloimmunization that potentially can cause rejection; however, if transfusion cannot be avoided, blood products should be leukoreduced and checked for CMV.[23]

Malignancy

The risk for malignancy is at most sites is far greater in renal transplant patients than it is in the general population. The most commonly occurring cancers in this population include those of the skin (melanoma, nonmelanoma, and Kaposi sarcoma), renal carcinomas, and non-Hodgkin lymphoma.[24] The risk of malignancy is directly proportional to the immunosuppressive load and time elapsed since transplant.[4]

Continued age-appropriate and gender-appropriate cancer screenings are of utmost importance, and skin cancer screenings should be performed every 6 months to a year by a dermatologist or experienced health care provider.[25]

Diabetes

Even patients without an underlying history of diabetes can develop new-onset diabetes after transplant. This is related to many issues, including predisposing factors like African American race, obesity, and family history as well as the diabetogenic side effects of immunosuppressive medications like glucocorticoids, CNIs, and mTOR inhibitors. Additionally, the functioning allograft is now more efficient and effective in clearing insulin from the body, and the allograft itself is gluconeogenic.[26] This propensity for glucose intolerance and diabetes in particular should be monitored closely in these patients in order to prevent the future complications of diabetes, including renal disease in the functioning allograft. Furthermore, there is evidence that renal transplant patients with diabetes may have higher rates of allograft rejection long-term.[27] Transplant patients should be screened regularly for diabetes with fasting blood glucose levels or hemoglobin A_{1c} levels. Treatment is similar to that of patients without a renal transplant, including the use of oral agents or subcutaneous insulin to control glucose levels appropriately.

Cardiovascular Disease

Cardiovascular disease (CVD) is the major cause of death in renal transplant patients, with studies attributing 50% to 60% of deaths in this population directly to CVD.[28] Contributing factors include diabetes, as described previously; hypertension; hyperlipidemia; and the side effects from immunosuppressive medications, especially the long-term use of glucocorticoids and sirolimus.[4] Each of these contributing factors should be monitored carefully and treated aggressively.

Hypertension in renal transplant patients is multifactorial as well, potentially stemming from rejection activity in the allograft, native kidney disease, CNI nephrotoxicity, or renal artery stenosis caused by an end-to-end anastomosis during the original transplant surgery. No matter the cause, renal transplant patients should be treated with calcium channel blockers or ACE inhibitors to a goal blood pressure of 120 to 130 mm Hg/70 to 80 mm Hg[4] in order to lower their risk for CVD.

SUMMARY

Patients with a functioning renal allograft represent a growing population that requires not only ongoing monitoring of renal function but also surveillance and treatment of potential complications and transplant-related conditions. Primary care providers can work closely with nephrologists to ensure that these patients protect their allograft and stay vigilant to other threats to their health, including infection, malignancy, and CVD. Such multidisciplinary care can help renal transplant patients maintain their quality of life.

DISCLOSURE

The authors have nothing to disclose.

REFERENCES

1. Port FK, Wolfe RA, Mauger EA, et al. Comparison of survival probabilities for dialysis patients vs cadaveric renal transplant recipients. JAMA 1993;270(11):1339.

2. Hart A, Smith JM, Skeans MA, et al. OPTN/SRTR 2018 Annual Data Report: Kidney. Am J Transplant 2020;20(S1):20–130.
3. Bunnapradist S, Danovitch GM. Evaluation of adult kidney transplant candidates. Am J Kidney Dis 2007;50(5):890.
4. Azzi J, Milford EL, Sayegh MH, et al. Transplantation in the treatment of renal failure. In: Jameson J, Fauci AS, Kasper DL, et al, editors. Harrison's Principles of internal medicine. 20th edition;2018. New York: McGraw-Hill.
5. Leung N, Lager DJ, Gertz MA, et al. Long-term outcome of renal transplantation in light-chain deposition disease. Am J Kidney Dis 2004;43(1):147.
6. Dobbels F, Vanhaecke J, Dupont L, et al. Pretransplant predictors of posttransplant adherence and clinical outcome: an evidence base for pretransplant psychosocial screening. Transplantation 2009;87(10):1497.
7. Gruessner AC, Dunn DL, Gruessner RG. Transplantation. In: Brunicardi F, Andersen DK, Billiar TR, et al, editors. Schwartz's principles of surgery. 11th edition;2019. New York: McGraw-Hill.
8. Port FK, Dykstra DM, Merion RM, et al. Trends and results for organ donation and transplantation in the United States, 2004. Am J Transplant 2005;5(4 Pt 2):843.
9. Gordon SM, LaRosa SP, Kalmadi S, et al. Should prophylaxis for Pneumocystis carinii pneumonia in solid organ transplant recipients ever be discontinued? Clin Infect Dis 1999;28(2):240.
10. Kotton CN, Kumar D, Caliendo AM, et al. The Third International Consensus Guidelines on the Management of Cytomegalovirus in Solid-organ Transplantation. Transplantation 2018;102(6):900.
11. Kidney Disease: Improving Global Outcomes (KDIGO) Transplant Work Group. KDIGO clinical practice guideline for the care of kidney transplant recipients. Am J Transplant 2009;9(Suppl 3):S1.
12. Hart A, Smith JM, Skeans MA, et al. Kidney. Am J Transplant 2016;16(Suppl 2):11.
13. Voora S, Adey D. Management of kidney transplant recipients by general nephrologists: Core Curriculum 2019. Am J Kidney Dis 2019;73(6):866–79.
14. Schimmer BP, Funder W. Adrenocorticotropic hormone, adrenal steroids, and the adrenal cortex. In: Brunton LL, Hilal-Dandan R, Knollmann BC, editors. Goodman & Gilman's: the pharmacological basis of therapeutics. 13th edition;2017. New York: McGraw-Hill.
15. Webster AC, Lee VW, Chapman JR, et al. Target of rapamycin inhibitors (TOR-I; sirolimus and everolimus) for primary immunosuppression in kidney transplant recipients. Cochrane Database Syst Rev 2006;(2):CD004290.
16. Zaltzman JS, Nash M, Chiu R, et al. The benefits of renin-angiotensin blockade in renal transplant recipients with biopsy-proven allograft nephropathy. Nephrol Dial Transplant 2004;19(4):940.
17. Screening of donor and recipient prior to solid organ transplantation. Am J Transplant 2004;4(Suppl 10):10.
18. Mularoni A, Bertani A, Vizzini G, et al. Outcome of transplantation using organs from donors infected or colonized with carbapenem-resistant gram-negative bacteria. Am J Transplant 2015;15(10):2674.
19. Finberg RW, Fingeroth JD. Infections in transplant recipients. In: Jameson J, Fauci AS, Kasper DL, et al, editors. Harrison's principles of internal medicine. 20th edition;2018. New York: McGraw-Hill.
20. Randhawa PS, Finkelstein S, Scantlebury V, et al. Human polyoma virus-associated interstitial nephritis in the allograft kidney. Transplantation 1999; 67(1):103.

21. Nikkel LE, Mohan S, Zhang A, et al. Reduced fracture risk with early corticosteroid withdrawal after kidney transplant. Am J Transplant 2012;12(3):649–59.

22. Van Loo A, Vanholder R, Bernaert P, et al. Recombinant human erythropoietin corrects anaemia during the first weeks after renal transplantation: a randomized prospective study. Nephrol Dial Transplant 1996;11(9):1815.

23. Triulzi DJ. Specialized transfusion support for solid organ transplantation. Curr Opin Hematol 2002;9(6):527.

24. Kasiske BL, Snyder JJ, Gilbertson DT, et al. Cancer after kidney transplantation in the United States. Am J Transplant 2004;4(6):905.

25. EBPG Expert Group on Renal Transplantation. European best practice guidelines for renal transplantation. Section IV: Long-term management of the transplant recipient. IV.6.2. Cancer risk after renal transplantation. Skin cancers: prevention and treatment. Nephrol Dial Transplant 2002;17(Suppl 4):31.

26. Gerich JE, Meyer C, Woerle HJ, et al. Renal Gluconeogenesis: Its importance in human glucose homeostasis. Diabetes Care 2001;24(2):382–91.

27. Schiel R, Heinrich S, Steiner T, et al. Long-term prognosis of patients after kidney transplantation: a comparison of those with or without diabetes mellitus. Nephrol Dial Transplant 2005;20(3):611.

28. Ojo AO. Cardiovascular complications after renal transplantation and their prevention. Transplantation 2006;82(5):603.

UNITED STATES POSTAL SERVICE ®

Statement of Ownership, Management, and Circulation
(All Periodicals Publications Except Requester Publications)

1. Publication Title	2. Publication Number	3. Filing Date
PRIMARY CARE: CLINICS IN OFFICE PRACTICE	044 – 690	9/18/2020

4. Issue Frequency	5. Number of Issues Published Annually	6. Annual Subscription Price
MAR, JUN, SEP, DEC	4	$253.00

7. Complete Mailing Address of Known Office of Publication (Not printer) (Street, city, county, state, and ZIP+4®)

ELSEVIER INC.
230 Park Avenue, Suite 800
New York, NY 10169

Contact Person
Malathi Samayan

Telephone (Include area code)
91-44-4299-4507

8. Complete Mailing Address of Headquarters or General Business Office of Publisher (Not printer)

ELSEVIER INC.
230 Park Avenue, Suite 800
New York, NY 10169

9. Full Names and Complete Mailing Addresses of Publisher, Editor, and Managing Editor (Do not leave blank)

Publisher (Name and complete mailing address)

DOLORES MELONI, ELSEVIER INC.
1600 JOHN F KENNEDY BLVD. SUITE 1800
PHILADELPHIA, PA 19103-2899

Editor (Name and complete mailing address)

KATERINA HEIDHAUSEN, ELSEVIER INC.
1600 JOHN F KENNEDY BLVD. SUITE 1800
PHILADELPHIA, PA 19103-2899

Managing Editor (Name and complete mailing address)

PATRICK MANLEY, ELSEVIER INC.
1600 JOHN F KENNEDY BLVD. SUITE 1800
PHILADELPHIA, PA 19103-2899

10. Owner (Do not leave blank. If the publication is owned by a corporation, give the name and address of the corporation immediately followed by the names and addresses of all stockholders owning or holding 1 percent or more of the total amount of stock. If not owned by a corporation, give the names and addresses of the individual owners. If owned by a partnership or other unincorporated firm, give its name and address as well as those of each individual owner. If the publication is published by a nonprofit organization, give its name and address.)

Full Name	Complete Mailing Address
WHOLLY OWNED SUBSIDIARY OF REED/ELSEVIER, US HOLDINGS	1600 JOHN F KENNEDY BLVD. SUITE 1800 PHILADELPHIA, PA 19103-2899

11. Known Bondholders, Mortgagees, and Other Security Holders Owning or Holding 1 Percent or More of Total Amount of Bonds, Mortgages, or Other Securities. If none, check box ▶ ☐ None

Full Name	Complete Mailing Address
N/A	

12. Tax Status (For completion by nonprofit organizations authorized to mail at nonprofit rates) (Check one)
The purpose, function, and nonprofit status of this organization and the exempt status for federal income tax purposes:
☒ Has Not Changed During Preceding 12 Months
☐ Has Changed During Preceding 12 Months (Publisher must submit explanation of change with this statement)

PS Form **3526**, July 2014 [Page 1 of 4 (see instructions page 4)] PSN: 7530-01-000-9931   PRIVACY NOTICE: See our privacy policy on www.usps.com.

13. Publication Title		14. Issue Date for Circulation Data Below
PRIMARY CARE: CLINICS IN OFFICE PRACTICE		JULY 2020

15. Extent and Nature of Circulation			Average No. Copies Each Issue During Preceding 12 Months	No. Copies of Single Issue Published Nearest to Filing Date
a. Total Number of Copies (Net press run)			88	67
b. Paid Circulation (By Mail and Outside the Mail)	(1)	Mailed Outside-County Paid Subscriptions Stated on PS Form 3541 (Include paid distribution above nominal rate, advertiser's proof copies, and exchange copies)	42	35
	(2)	Mailed In-County Paid Subscriptions Stated on PS Form 3541 (Include paid distribution above nominal rate, advertiser's proof copies, and exchange copies)	0	0
	(3)	Paid Distribution Outside the Mails Including Sales Through Dealers and Carriers, Street Vendors, Counter Sales, and Other Paid Distribution Outside USPS®	14	8
	(4)	Paid Distribution by Other Classes of Mail Through the USPS (e.g., First-Class Mail®)	0	0
c. Total Paid Distribution (Sum of 15b (1), (2), (3), and (4))		▶	56	43
d. Free or Nominal Rate Distribution (By Mail and Outside the Mail)	(1)	Free or Nominal Rate Outside-County Copies included on PS Form 3541	16	7
	(2)	Free or Nominal Rate In-County Copies Included on PS Form 3541	0	0
	(3)	Free or Nominal Rate Copies Mailed at Other Classes Through the USPS (e.g. First-Class Mail)	0	0
	(4)	Free or Nominal Rate Distribution Outside the Mail (Carriers or other means)	16	7
e. Total Free or Nominal Rate Distribution (Sum of 15d (1), (2), (3) and (4))		▶	16	7
f. Total Distribution (Sum of 15c and 15e)		▶	72	50
g. Copies not Distributed (See Instructions to Publishers #4 (page #3))		▶	16	17
h. Total (Sum of 15f and g)		▶	88	67
i. Percent Paid (15c divided by 15f times 100)			77.77%	86%

* If you are claiming electronic copies, go to line 16 on page 3. If you are not claiming electronic copies, skip to line 17 on page 3.

16. Electronic Copy Circulation	Average No. Copies Each Issue During Preceding 12 Months	No. Copies of Single Issue Published Nearest to Filing Date
a. Paid Electronic Copies	▶	
b. Total Paid Print Copies (Line 15c) + Paid Electronic Copies (Line 16a)	▶	
c. Total Print Distribution (Line 15f) + Paid Electronic Copies (Line 16a)	▶	
d. Percent Paid (Both Print & Electronic Copies) (16b divided by 16c × 100)	▶	

☒ I certify that 50% of all my distributed copies (electronic and print) are paid above a nominal price.

17. Publication of Statement of Ownership

☒ If the publication is a general publication, publication of this statement is required. Will be printed ☐ Publication not required.
in the DECEMBER 2020 issue of this publication.

18. Signature and Title of Editor, Publisher, Business Manager, or Owner		Date
Malathi Samayan - Distribution Controller	*Malathi Samayan*	9/18/2020

I certify that all information furnished on this form is true and complete. I understand that anyone who furnishes false or misleading information on this form or who omits material or information requested on the form may be subject to criminal sanctions (including fines and imprisonment) and/or civil sanctions (including civil penalties).

PS Form **3526**, July 2014 (Page 3 of 4)   PRIVACY NOTICE: See our privacy policy on www.usps.com.

Printed and bound by CPI Group (UK) Ltd, Croydon, CR0 4YY

03/10/2024

01040401-0017